HOFFER'S LAWS OF
NATURAL
NUTRITION

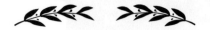

QUARRY PRESS
BODY•MIND•SPIRIT

Vitamin B-3 and Schizophrenia:
Discovery, Recovery, Controversy
by DR. ABRAM HOFFER

Vitamin C and Cancer:
Discovery, Recovery, Controversy
by DR. ABRAM HOFFER

Seeds in the Wilderness:
Profiles of World Religious Leaders
by MARTY GERVAIS

Cotapaxi Visions:
Travels in Ecuador
by JOE FISHER

Transcendental Anarchy:
Confessions of a Metaphysical Tourist
by LESLEY CHOYCE

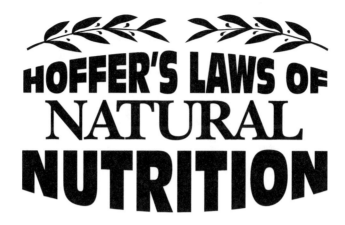

HOFFER'S LAWS OF NATURAL NUTRITION

A GUIDE TO EATING WELL FOR PURE HEALTH

Abram Hoffer M.D.

QUARRY PRESS
BODY•MIND•SPIRIT

Dedicated to Fran Fuller, for without her secretarial help this book could not have been written, and for her dedication, interest, and care of our patients, which has made my office so comfortable for them. Rarely do they leave my office without saying good-bye to Fran, and often they appear more disappointed when she is away, than if I were away.

Thanks, Fran.

The nutritional, medical, and health information presented in this book is based on the research, training, and personal experiences of the author, and is true and complete to the best of the author's knowledge. However, this book is intended only as an informative guide for those wishing to know more about nutrition. It is not intended to replace or countermand the advice given to you by your physician. Because each person and each situation is unique, the publisher urges the reader to check with a qualified health professional before using any procedure where there is any question as to its appropriateness.

The publisher does not advocate the use of any particular supplement program, but believes that the information presented in this book should be available to the public. Because there is always some risk involved, the author and publisher are not responsible for any adverse effects or consequences resulting from the use of any of the suggestions in this book. Please feel free to consult a physician or other qualified health professional. It is a sign of wisdom, not cowardice, to seek a second or third opinion.

The publisher acknowledges the financial assistance of The Canada Council, the Ontario Arts Council, and the Department of Canadian Heritage.

Canadian Cataloguing in Publication Data

Hoffer, Abram, 1917–
   Hoffer's Laws of natural nutrition : a guide to eating well for pure health

ISBN 1-55082-095-8

   1. Diet therapy. 2. Diet and disease. 3. Nutrition.
I. Title

RA784.H64 1994   615.8'54   C94-900284-4

Printed and bound in Canada by Best Book Manufacturers inc, Toronto, Ontario.

Published by Quarry Press Inc.,
P.O. Box 1061, Kingston, Ontario K7L 4Y5.

CONTENTS

I
THE TWENTIETH-CENTURY DILEMMA IN HEALTH

II
THE HEALTH COSTS OF THE HIGH-TECH DIET

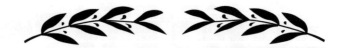

III
THE HEALTH BENEFITS
OF A NATURAL DIET

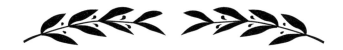

IV
THE TWENTY-FIRST CENTURY
DIRECTION IN HEALTH

V
THE NUTRIENT CONTENT
OF COMMON FOODS

VI
SOURCES OF INFORMATION
ON GOOD NUTRITION

I

THE TWENTIETH-CENTURY
DILEMMA IN HEALTH

BEYOND
THE HIGH-TECH DIET

⁜

The three basic elements of good health are our genetic inheritance, our education, and our chemical environment, of which food and how we use it to construct our diet is a major component. We cannot yet change our genetic inheritance, although this is an objective pursued by some scientists, but we can and must know how health is connected with food and nutrition so that we can extract the maximum benefit from available food and nutrients. And we must pass this information on to our children at home and in our schools beginning with the earliest grades.

> **LAW**
>
> *The three basic elements of good health are our genetic inheritance, our education, and our chemical environment, of which food and how we use it to construct our diet is a major component.*

Before the development of food technology, not counting the introduction of fire and cooking, we only needed to know what foods were safe and which ones would make us sick or kill us. This information was developed by personal experiences passed on by example and instruction to our offspring. We did not have to depend upon reading and lectures. Fortunately, we did have good instincts based upon our sense of taste, smell, and touch. These are the senses

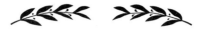

that guide animals in their selection of food. Potential plant or animal food which did not taste good was avoided. Usually this meant these products were too bitter. Foods that taste bland, salty, or sweet were preferred and as a rule are not poisonous. If any food made us sick, this would soon be recognized and thereafter avoided. We used other clues, such as the appearance and the tactile feel of the food, to decide whether or not to eat the food. From the small number of foods which were safe it was normal healthy practice to eat what was available without knowing anything about the composition of those foods. These were all whole foods, which in themselves were well balanced and which could maintain health. Whole wheat can nourish animals for long periods of time, while white flour will soon cause the same animals to die if this is their only food source.

Modern high-tech food processing, however, has robbed us of the use of our senses in determining whether a food is or is not good for us. Modern foods are designed to appeal to the senses. Visually they are packaged in appealing containers and painted with interesting colors. They are usually sweet, some much more than others, contain some salt (usually too much), and are thus made attractive to the mouth. These cosmetic attributes are given to all the overly processed foods, ranging from those that will make one sick because they are so inadequate in their nutrient composition to those that are more nourishing. It is no longer possible to depend upon our senses to determine how nourishing food will be. For this reason we now have to depend upon our education to select foods that will serve us as well as they did before these high-tech processes became so common. This will be very difficult because an enormous advertising

Modern high-tech food processing has robbed us of the use of our senses in determining whether a food is or is not good for us.

LAW

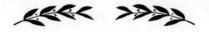

industry drives home the message that all these foods are good for you. They emphasize that sweet is healthy. Public education will have to displace all that commercial advertising. I would recommend that advertising for junk foods ought to be placed in the same category as advertising for tobacco, alcohol, and addicting drugs.

Modern high quality nutrition depends upon the combination of good nutritional education and an adequate supply of foods so that the education can be applied to the selection of a healthy diet. But I do not think that the education needs to be of the caliber required of nutritionists, dietitians, and physicians. The majority of people do not have to know the amount of vitamins present in foods, the amount of fat or carbohydrate. They do not have to be so skillful with nutrients that they can construct a diet entirely derived from the 50 or so nutrients. It is enough to know which of the food products available to them are healthy and which are not. This book is written for the majority of people who do not want to spend much time on food tables but who wish to have a few simple guidelines which they can follow and which will ensure that they will become healthy and remain well.

The loss of our senses as a good guide for selecting our food is the main reason for what I shall call the twentieth-century dilemma in the field of disease and health. Stated briefly, the dilemma is the close parallel development between the rise in the amount of chronic disease and the improvement in the technology of medicine and surgery. Medicine and surgery have made enormous strides in curing a number of diseases such as infections, in preventing

LAW

The loss of our senses as a good guide for selecting our food is the main reason for what I shall call the twentieth-century dilemma in the field of disease and health. Stated briefly, the dilemma is the close parallel development between the rise in the amount of chronic disease and the improvement in the technology of medicine and surgery.

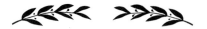

deficiency disease such as scurvy or beri beri, and in surgical and anesthetic methods for doing superb surgery with a minimum of pain and other discomfort. In fact it was commonly believed when I graduated in medicine in 1949 that we were on the threshold of the wonder era in medicine when we could look forward to a society free of disease and enjoying an optimum state of health. The antibiotics had at last been fully accepted, the corticosteroid drugs such as cortisone and ACTH were curing almost everything, and surgery was being rapidly perfected. The financial development of government run health plans in countries like Canada depended upon the assumptions that the number of people requiring care and treatment would decrease as a result of new drug treatment and surgical methods. But parallel to the remarkable advances in medicine and surgery we have seen an equally remarkable increase in chronic cardiovascular disease, cancer, diabetes, and so on.

During my adult years I have seen an enormous increase in the number of people who become sick. In 1950 when I started my education in psychiatry we saw very few children with learning and behavioral disorders. We did see children who could not learn and who were said to be retarded, but the combination of hyperactivity and learning disorder so common today was very rare. I believe that pediatricians who can still remember what their practices were like in the 1950s will support this conclusion. Today these problem children are so numerous many pediatricians look upon this as normal behavior which they will outgrow. Breast cancer has increased from 1 in 20 women to 1 in 9 women in the past 20 years, and may still be increasing. In the United States a few years ago there were 750,000 cardiovascular deaths, 164,300 cerebrovascular deaths, and 465,000 cancer deaths. I have estimated that every second Canadian has one or more chronic disease. This figure is easily arrived at by adding up the number who are obese and suffer the consequences of the diseases caused by their low fiber, high sugar

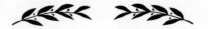

diet; the alcoholics and addicts; the mentally sick, especially the Alzheimers sufferers and schizophrenics; the victims of muscular degenerative diseases and some of the modern plagues such as the viral influenzas and AIDS.

Obviously advances in drug research and surgical skill have not led to better health. Poor eating and nutritional ignorance have, however, led to an increase in chronic disease. The twentieth-century dilemma is caused by the combination of the persuasive power of high-tech food processing industry and the poor quality of the nutritional education given to our children. It follows that there will be no solution to the problem of chronic illness until we become aware that only by the selection of those foods which can nourish us properly will there ever be a decrease in the growth of the chronic disease industry.

Yet some physicians and public health officials persist in talking about the overall state of improvement of our health, using the fact that many more people today reach retirement age than did people 100 years ago. The real test of general health is not how many reach the age of 65 but how closely can we push the average age of death to the theoretical limit of 110 to 120 years. We have improved a little. A man age 55 in 1900 could expect to live another 17 years on the average. Today that same man can expect to live about 20 more years. Our grandparents could expect almost the same additional years of life as we can.

J.D. Beasley and J.J. Swift in their classic book *The Kellogg Report: The Impact of Nutrition, Environment and Lifestyle on the Health of Americans* observe that "adults today may be living a couple of years longer than our ancestors, but we're still being cut down before our time." We are not "doing better than ever"; we are simply being killed off by disease at slightly later points in our lives. The irony is that these diseases are a product of our own living patterns. To quote former U.S. Health, Education, and Welfare (HEW) Secretary Joseph Califano, "I can compress what we have learned about the

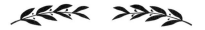

causes of these modern killers in three summarizing sentences: We are killing ourselves by our own careless habits. We are killing ourselves by carelessly polluting the environment. We are killing ourselves by permitting harmful social conditions to persist — conditions like poverty, hunger, and ignorance — which destroy health, especially in infants and children." He also reported that "while death from the major acute infections and diseases plummeted between 1900 and 1970, the proportion of mortality from major chronic disease, such as heart disease, cancer and stroke, increased more than 250 percent."

My reason for writing this book is to provide the kind of information I think most people want so that they can select intelligently those foods which are good for them, but not necessarily for everyone. This will not be a panacea diet in the sense that one diet will be good for every person. It will not be a high protein or high carbohydrate diet, a low fat or vegetarian, an acid base or blood type diet.

Diet books are now popular and have often become best sellers. I have no quarrel with any diet books, even with those which are panacea diets, except when these diets are prescribed to be followed by everyone. They ignore the most important principle or law of nutrition: we are all different. They probably were discovered by people who found out that when they altered their diet they felt very much better. They naturally assumed that if it helped them, it must be helpful for everyone. They would then tell their family and friends and some of them would also feel much better. For example, simply advising every one to discontinue all dairy products or all wheat products will make a

> *Diet books have been very popular and have often become best sellers. I have no quarrel with any diet books, even with those which are panacea diets, except when these diets are prescribed to be followed by everyone. They ignore the most important principle or law of nutrition: we are all different.*

LAW

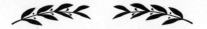

sizable proportion of that group feel much better, for allergies to these foods are so common. The others who had responded would then by word of mouth impart the good news to their friends and eventually the originator would feel that the message is important and ought to be publicized widely in a book, pamphlets, and so on. People who tried that diet and either did not respond or got worse would likely not tell their friends about it and so there would be a large number of supporters and very few critics. But these diets ignore individuality and they ignore the presence of food allergies or toxic reactions.

The diet I recommend will be discovered by each person in a scientific way, a diet which is therefore individualized, or tailor made, and which once discovered will need only minor adjustments with changing circumstances. It will be a panacea *method* which can be applied by almost everyone. I have found it very useful in advising thousands of my patients how to determine their own optimum diet and it has been one which can be mastered fairly easily. After that patients are armed against the cure-all diets appearing on the scene at regular intervals and they are able to maintain their health with little need to consult physicians.

TOWARDS A NATURAL DIET

v

There are many people who are well and therefore do not need to modify their diet. They, obviously, have found the diet to which they are adapted. Any modification of their diet would likely make them worse if it were continued for a long time. So the question is, how can you find out for yourself if you have good health or whether your health can be made better by changing the food consumed? There are two sides to this question, one short term, the other long term. Are you well now? Will you be well many years from now? In my view the state of health ought to be so good that there is no deterioration towards the end of one's life.

Most people know when they are in good health. They are able to feel rested and relaxed after six to eight hours of sleep, they awaken in the morning feeling well and looking forward to the day. They enjoy the food they eat. At work or at home they have enough energy to do what they want to do and they do not become excessively tired even in the evening. They will carry on with the day without becoming excessively sleepy or tired in the mid morning or mid afternoon, an indication that food allergies are present. During the day and later on at home they will remain in good humor, free of depression, unless there is something which would depress any other normal person such as the loss of an idea, loss of a job, death of a friend or family member,

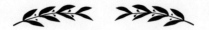

or any other major disappointment. When they do feel sad, this will in time clear as it does for normal people. They will not suffer prolonged deep depression long after the event which precipitated it has passed. They will enjoy their work or profession, or if it cannot be enjoyed, they will tolerate it and find other activities to make up for what they are not getting from their work. They will make decisions which are rational most of the time. They are able to deal with stress. When they get sick, they recover in fewer days than do most people who are not well. If this is their state of health, they are in my opinion in good health.

I use four main criteria for evaluating the state of health of my patients:

1. Are they free of signs and symptoms of ill-health or disease?
2. Are they getting on reasonably well with their family?
3. Are they getting on reasonably well with the community?
4. Are they working, either at home or on the job?

I define work as any activity that a person does, whether or not they are being paid to do it. If my patients fail to achieve even one of these four main points, I do not consider them well.

To evaluate your own health you should consider the following questions:

1. Do you have enough energy to do what you want to do or are you suffering from too much fatigue? Are you tired too much of the time, especially when it is not appropriate to be tired?
2. Is your mood fairly stable with swings into depression or cheerfulness appropriate to events

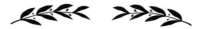

and considered appropriate by other people in similar circumstances?

3. Do you have symptoms which indicate you might be suffering from any disease?

If you do not have any known condition, you should then determine whether you are suffering from one of the many forms of malnutrition, from a defect arising from poor diet, from a vitamin or mineral deficiency, or from any one of the nutrient dependencies.

If you are well, not much needs to be done. Either you are already on a good diet to which you have been adapted, or you have such a marvelous constitution and biochemistry that you can remain well even on a less perfect diet. Your only concern is for the future. It would be wise to tighten up the diet by following the nutritional laws and principles described in this book and to supplement this by taking the optimum amount of vitamin C and a good B-complex vitamin preparation. Many people are surprised after they have been following this vitamin program for several months how much better they feel.

Many years ago a high-school teacher came to me with his identical twin schizophrenic brother. His brother had been ill for many years and was not able to work. I prescribed vitamin B-3 and vitamin C for him and arranged to see him regularly to follow his progress. Several months later the "normal" brother asked me whether he could take the same vitamins. I assured him that he could. He had seen great improvement in his schizophrenic twin and wondered what the supplements might do for him. A few months later he told he that he had always considered himself well, but when he realized how much better he felt on the vitamins, he knew that he had not been as well as he had thought he was. I have seen the same realization in families where the mother and/or wife became my patient. I would advise her to follow a good diet, usually by eliminating sugar and junk and very often milk plus any other food she might be allergic to. I would outline which vitamins she ought to take. Very often the husband, who was well, did not want to give up sweets and desserts, and my patient did not want to deprive him of these. However, after many months of preparing two sets of meals, one for herself and one for the rest of the family, she would decide to place the whole family on her diet, primarily because she was now well. In most cases she would gradually decrease the sweets program and eventually would have the whole family on her diet. I would then hear from her how much healthier the whole family was. The husband was more energetic, less irritable, and more relaxed. If the husband was with her, he would cheerfully admit the change in himself and how he had resisted changing. My patient would often tell me the whole family had had the flu or a severe cold and she had remained well. In the past she had developed the same virus infections as they had.

LAW | *Every person, no matter how well they feel, can determine very easily how well they really are by placing themselves on the natural diet recommended in this book, with or without supplements.*

Every person, no matter how well they feel, can determine very easily how well they really are by placing themselves on the natural diet recommended in this book, with or without supplements.

If you are not well, the first step is to have a medical check up from your doctor, especially if you suspect you are experiencing the symptoms of any disease. Anything you and your doctor find must be corrected. After that you should follow a procedure of improving your diet and adding the correct supplements. It is desirable to do this with medical supervision, but you may find it very difficult to find a physician or nutritionist able to advise you. If you cannot find a physician, read everything you can about how to do so.

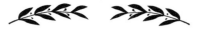

To discover your optimum diet, I recommend the following 4-step program for pure health:

Step 1. Eliminate all the junk from your diet, especially all the free sugars, and any food you suspect you might be allergic to. Add vitamin C 1 gram after each meal. Stay on this diet for at least one month. If by then you feel well, this is your diet. If you are not any better or have gained only a little, examine your diet again for other possible food allergies, including allergies to dairy products and processed protein. Then eliminate them and carry on for another month. If you cannot find any other food allergies, go to step 2.

Step 2. Add a good vitamin B-complex tablet or one of the stress tablets. I like the B-complex 50 or 100 preparations. You can take as many as you wish but in most cases 1 to 3 tablets per day will be adequate. These all contain riboflavin or Vitamin B-2, which will color the urine yellow. This is a good test whether or not the vitamins are being absorbed in the gastro-intestinal tract. Stay on this program for several months. If you have not reached the state of well being you want, then start to add other individual vitamins, minerals, and fatty acids. The main objective of this book is to describe these nutrients and how to use them well enough so that you can use them with safety. All these nutrients are compatible and can be taken together, usually with food in the stomach. Nutrients are compatible with all medication and with each other.

Step 3. For the rest of your life keep reviewing both your diet and the supplements you are taking because requirements change with age, with sickness, with degree of stress. There is only one way of knowing and that is to be alert to the need to the changes in you and to the changes you must make in your diet. There is a constant need to maintain the adjustment

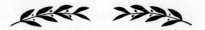

between your needs and the food you eat.

Step 4. If you are still not well, you probably have very serious problems and will have to consult specialists in the field of orthomolecular medicine, the field of medicine I founded with such colleagues as Linus Pauling, Humphry Osmond, and Wilfrid and Evan Shute.

From this book, you should be able to determine if you are suffering from one of the many forms of malnutrition, from a health defect arising from poor diet, from a vitamin or mineral deficiency, or from any one of the nutrient dependencies. You should be able to discover a diet which will lead you out of the twentieth-century dilemma in nutrition into a new age of pure health.

II

THE HEALTH COSTS
OF THE HIGH-TECH DIET

THE JUNK FOOD
ERA

᭢

VOMIT REFLEX

The reason why we should eat for the best health is so obvious it should not have to be restated. Nature has spent millions of years perfecting animals and plants so that they can extract the best from other plants and animals which make up our food. The primary objective of life is to perpetuate itself; survival is absolutely essential, at least until the species has passed reproductive age and the genes of the elderly are no longer needed for species survival. Animals are therefore endowed with senses which help them to identify potential food and with enough logic to decide when they should try to obtain these foods. These foods must be harmless and also must be nourishing if the animal is to live and reproduce.

But how can animals decide which foods are the ones best for them? Obviously they have done a better job of this than we have in the modern age of high-tech food. They have done this by judging the quality of the food by the impact it has on their health. The effect of eating the food may be immediate, within a few minutes or hours, or it may require weeks or months before it becomes evident. The immediate effect of toxic food has been examined by scientists who have found that there is a powerful gag and

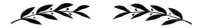

vomiting reflex. When animals eat something which is highly toxic for them, and if it can be identified by its bad taste or by some other attribute, that animal will no longer eat that particular food.

Attempts have been made to manipulate this natural reflex to control the appetite of natural predators for farm animals. Lithium salts have been placed in sheep's meat and scattered in areas where natural predators live. The encounter between the animal, a fox or coyote, has been filmed. The animal ate the meat with relish but shortly after was made violently ill with retching and vomiting. Thereafter that animal would no longer eat sheep's meat. When the same animal found other sheep's meat, it would turn away apparently in disgust. It was hoped that this would produce the same aversion to living sheep as it had to their poisoned flesh. Conventional wisdom says that if you are going to poison rats, you had better put in enough poison so that they are killed the first time. The survivors will not eat the same bait again if it can be identified by taste or smell or some other attribute.

Human beings have the same survival reflex, though the creators of our modern high-tech foods have so successfully masked potentially poisonous products with flavors and other additives that this reflex is often delayed or deadened. Many years ago a mother brought two of her sons to see me. One was adopted. Both were seven years old, both suffered from severe hyperactivity, and both were having learning difficulties. I suspected that the amount of sugar and junk food they were eating was a factor and advised the two children and their mother that they should go onto a sugar free diet. The two children were horrified. One month later one child was well and the other remained as hyperactive as he had been before. The boy who was well had been following the diet, while the other refused to do so. He told me in no uncertain terms that he would never ever stop eating sugar and stamped his foot to emphasize his decision.

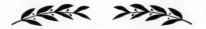

I then advised them to go on to plan B. They both asked me what was plan B, expecting something even worse. I asked them, would they follow the no sugar diet on week days if they could have all the junk they wanted on Saturday? They both agreed. When they came back after another month both boys were well. Their mother then told me what had happened.

In preparation for junk-food Saturday they had gone to a store. The boy who had been cooperative before was very upset because his brother was going to get all those sweets. His mother agreed he could also go onto the same program. But then the five other children in the family complained that they were being left out. Mother finally said the whole family could do so. The following Saturday one of the children became violently ill with nausea and vomiting after consuming sweets. Pretty soon every child in that family was sick with either headaches, nausea, or vomiting. After that the little boy who had been so determined he would never give up sweets told me, adamantly, that he would never ever eat sweets again.

This survival or vomiting reflex may be written as a rule or law of natural nutrition: Avoid any food which makes you sick or which is psychologically disgusting to you.

We use our senses to identify potentially offensive food and our experiences and beliefs determine whether we will vomit when we consume that food. Smell and taste are the most important senses involved in this survival reflex. Smell forewarns the person that the food may be toxic. Bad smelling foods are generally not liked unless long experience with that bad smell has convinced the person that the food is not toxic. This would apply to very ripe cheeses and other odoriferous foods. Smell warns one even when the

---

LAW *This survival or vomiting reflex may be written as a rule or law of natural nutrition: Avoid any food which makes you sick or which is psychologically disgusting to you.*

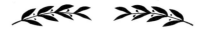

food is many feet away. Smell will of course also foretell that good food is available, if that smell is associated with food a person has enjoyed. If the food passes the odor test and is placed in one's mouth, taste becomes the next arbiter. But taste also depends to a large degree on the sense of smell. That is why people with plugged noses, with colds or allergies, will not have the same sense of taste as when they are well. In the same way people deficient in zinc will lose their ability to both taste and smell foods.

The four basic tastes are bitter, sour, salty, and sweet. Usually foods which are bitter are not liked. Alkaloids tend to taste bitter and they are poisonous. Animals have learned early on that these are best avoided. Plants defending themselves against being consumed will form these bitter tasting substances. Nicotine was developed by the tobacco plant to protect itself against predators, not for the enjoyment and destruction of people. The sour (acid) and salty tastes are accepted or rejected, depending on the concentrations of compounds present in the food and therefore on the intensity of the taste. Very sour foods will be rejected but lesser degrees of acidity may make the food very desirable. Many people love very sour pickles, for example. Excessive sourness is a warning sign to which people pay attention. The same applies to salty foods. Some love excessive amounts of salt. This is one of the factors in the current high incidence of high blood pressure and hypertension.

The almost universally liked taste is sweetness. These foods are usually safe to eat because they contain no bitter and poisonous compounds. There is an optimum concentration of the sugars which varies tremendously. Some love excessive amounts. It is not uncommon for many, especially alcoholics, to add enough sugar to their coffee to make it a saturated solution with crystals left in the bottom. Others cannot tolerate this much. People who have been on a sugar free or low sugar diet long enough generally develop a dislike for too much sweetness in their foods. I have not

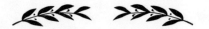

added sugar or sweetener to my drinks for 50 years. I could not drink coffee if it contained ¼ teaspoon of sugar; it would be cloyingly sweet for me. Foods which are bland are also acceptable and preferred by many. Bland foods include breads, potatoes, rice, all the cereals. A bland food can be consumed in large amounts without satiating the person and they can be used as carriers for other foods such as gravy, jam, and butter. When bland foods taste bitter or salty or sour, they will be quickly rejected unless it is known that products have been added to impart this quality to the food.

Almost all the overly processed foods contain sugar. The amount present in some foods will surprise many. Thus catsup contains 30 percent sugar. Some breakfast cereals have more sugar in them than do chocolate bars, containing over 50 percent sugar. The love for sweetness is so great it makes sugar the best addicting drug we have today. Overly processed food contains lots of sugar for the following reasons: (1) sugar masks the bland taste of overly processed foods which tend to remove the natural flavors of the original raw food; (2) it is addicting. If there are two competing pea soups made by different companies, the one with the most sugar in it will sell the best. There is an advantage to the bottom line if one can sell sugar in the product at the price of beans or peas when the price of sugar is low enough. There are a number of sugars. Food additives which end with "ose" are sugars, such as sucrose (table sugar), lactose (milk sugar), fructose, glucose, maltose, and so on. If companies want to avoid the intent of labeling laws, they will use several different sugars so that these sugars can be printed further from the beginning of the label. By law if sugar is the major ingredient, it must be listed first. If, however, one uses three different sugars, each one will be listed further on. It is thus possible to have a product which is 60 percent sugar but none of the sugars will appear first since individually these are not the major components. Sugar is the pervasive food additive, present in almost all processed food, which also

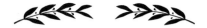

contains a number of other food additives to create "desirable" properties of taste, color, odor, consistency, stability, or emulsifiability. They are *not* added to enhance the nutritional quality of the food.

> *Once people see and feel the connection between what they eat and how they feel — once the original survival mechanism has been reactivated — there is very little further difficulty in following what I call the "No Sugar Law": Eliminate Foods with Sugar Additives from Your Diet.*

LAW

Indeed, food additives, especially sugar, can be harmful to good health. A person eating daily large amounts of sugar of one type or another when given an additional amount of sugar will not react adversely to it, but the sugar may be causing a large number of pathological reactions in the body that are chronic. Excessive eating of sugar causes sharp reactions in many people when they have become allergic to it. They will consume a quantity of sugar or even binge on it. This is followed by a feeling of well being which may last several hours, and this in turn is followed by a major or minor slump into depression and fatigue. I have seen patients who would go into a hypomanic state for three to four days after a sugar binge, followed by a major depression lasting many days. When they eat large amounts every day, this effect upon their mood is masked by the general ill health from which they suffer. In order to reactivate the connection between the intake of the substance and the reaction of the body, it is necessary to eliminate the product from that person's diet for at least five days, sometimes for up to one month. At the end of that time the immune system has recovered to the extent that if one then consumes the sugar there will be a sharp reaction. This will be apparent to the person and certainly to family members in close proximity. It is especially notable with children. Once people see and feel the connection between what they eat and how they feel — once the original survival mechanism

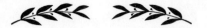

has been reactivated — there is very little further difficulty in following what I call the "No Sugar Law": Eliminate Foods with Sugar Additives from Your Diet.

Overly processed foods are rich not only in sugar but also in fats, salt, and other additives with xenobiotic or foreign flavors. It is important to make the final product taste and smell good but the original appetizing characteristics of the food are destroyed by the processing. The manufacturers therefore give a new flavor to that food by adding all these additives. Many people, I am sure, can only recognize the sensations of sweetness or saltiness. When they are placed upon a sugar free diet, which usually also removes the other additives, they will many months later remark how good other food tastes again, something they had forgotten over the years.

Foods to which an animal has not adapted or foods which contain toxins that do not kill immediately produce chronic ill health. An example would be the placing of arsenic in one's food in small amounts. Arsenic tastes sweet and is therefore not detectable by taste or smell. Over the weeks and months it will make the person quite ill. This was at one time a favorite method for poisoning enemies. These toxic or poisonous foods do not alarm the animal since there is no way the senses can alert them to the danger. But in the long run these foods will make the animals sick, they will not be able to reproduce, and eventually their genes will vanish. Chronic disease will make the animals less fit to survive and they will be eliminated by predators and by other forces from the environment. But these animals will not know what has been happening to them. Animals who have different likes and dislikes might by accident develop a dislike for those foods which would make them sick, and these animals would eventually take over from the other members of the species and become the dominant one. Thus genetics would also help in the survival process by helping animals avoid foods to which they are not adapted.

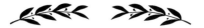

Modern high-tech food removes the natural ability of our senses to warn us about the lack of nutrition of the food because all these foods are made too sweet, too salty, and too flavorful with xenobiotic flavoring agents. This is why the majority of people have no idea that the food which they buy and which they consume does not nourish them and is mainly responsible for a large number of chronic diseases. Infants learn basic nutrition from their parents as they graduate from milk to solid foods as soon as their digestive apparatus is capable of dealing with them. They learn by observing what their parents eat and by eating food brought to them by their parents. They will also experiment with food tastes, avoiding the ones that taste too unusual or taste bitter. They will learn by being made sick by eating certain foods. But they will not draw the connection between taste and health when eating toxic food which has a low level of toxicity but which will make them just as sick over a period of months or years. Only from their parents, teachers, or doctors can they learn this connection and thus eliminate low level toxic food from their diet.

> *Modern high-tech food removes the natural ability of our senses to warn us about the lack of nutrition of the food because all these foods are made too sweet, too salty, and too flavorful with xenobiotic flavoring agents. This is why the majority of people have no idea that the food which they buy and which they consume does not nourish them and is mainly responsible for a large number of chronic diseases.*

LAW

Man has been pretty good at discovering the 100 or so different plants we can use as food from the many thousands of plants that could have been food but which are either poisonous, toxic, or not nourishing. Until the beginning of modern food technology about 10,000 years ago, we did pretty well. All the foods which were available culled from the much large total potential supply were nourishing. We did not have to worry about balanced diets, since all these

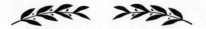

foods, no matter in what combination they were used, were inherently well balanced. The balance was destroyed from foods after the introduction of food technology, especially its development over the past 50 years. Until the dawn of agriculture we did not have to use our intellect to eat well. Our main problem was to obtain enough food. What was available was nutritious. We suffered food shortages and often starvation, and as we moved to colder climates began to suffer from annual epidemics of scurvy. Fruits and fresh vegetation were not available in those times. Today we have too much food. We no longer are worried about starvation in highly industrialized nations, but we now have a major problem deriving good nutrition from the depleted quality of our food. We live with an abundance of low quality food which we eat indiscriminately and which makes most of us chronically sick. We have arrived at the time in our evolution when we can no longer depend upon our senses and have to depend upon our intelligence and knowledge to select only those foods to which we have been adapted and which will keep us well as long as we are alive. The major problem with modern food technology is that it has destroyed our senses as good indicators for what foods are safe and nutritious and for what foods are not.

RAW, COOKED, REFINED, AND PROCESSED FOODS

Our modern high-tech diets have been developing over the past ten thousand years but the pace of change has accelerated sharply over the past 50 years. We have the same genetic structure our ancestors had ten thousand years ago but the food supply today is totally different from what it was then. The change in our food supply has been so rapid that it has been impossible for evolution to keep pace. Most of the diseases endemic to high-tech societies arise from this maladjustment between our long-developed adaptation to our environment and our contemporary nutritional

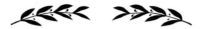

habits, between ourselves and our food.

Our relationships to our food can be divided into four major eras. Each succeeding era is shorter than the preceding one. The last one, the era of "junk" food, is probably 100 years old, merely a second in the time required for our culture to develop. Each era represents an accelerated transformation of our diet, completely outstripping our ability to adapt.

The "Raw" Era

During this era man must have had the same foods as any other primates. We were hunters and gatherers, depending primarily on vegetable food and supplementing this with animals foods which could be caught. It is unlikely we lived in the cold polar regions since fire had not been discovered. This means we had access to vegetables year round and so did not suffer from spring scurvy so common more recently in Europe. Starvation was more of a problem than malnutrition. Obesity must have been extremely rare.

The "Cooked" Era

With the discovery of fire, man began to cook food, especially the animals that could be dismembered and cut up with newly-discovered cutting utensils or knives. The advent of cooking was on the whole beneficial to health. It made it easier to digest certain vegetables and softened animal food, thus requiring less work in eating. It also destroyed insects and parasites, thus decreasing infectious diseases. I do not think it made food more palatable, for palatability is a matter of experience. Excluding the bitter tasting foods, people enjoy food which tastes like food they have enjoyed in their infancy and youth. People who are used to eating raw, fresh meat will continue to enjoy this meat. We who are accustomed to cooked meat in appearance, texture, and taste find raw meat repulsive. But it cannot be concluded that cooking has made our food more palatable. I recall seeing a

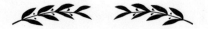

documentary describing the habits of native people in the South Pacific. Two teen-aged girls were walking along the beach. Suddenly one girl pounced on the sand, drew out a long wriggling worm, and with obvious relish ate it on the spot, much as a North American teenager might enjoy a hamburger or an ice cream cone.

There are many disadvantages to cooking. Heat alters the natural state of food and makes it less nutritious, less able to support life. Proteins are denatured. Their structure is altered so that enzymes designed to digest living protein tissue now must work on denatured tissue. Amino acids recombine into new peptides which may be harder to digest, or they may combine with sugar to form brown substances. The outside of a broiled or fried steak or a roast is brown for this reason. Unsaturated fats are oxidized by heat and essential fatty acids are destroyed. Starches are made more digestible but sugars are oxidized. Heat labile vitamins, such as vitamins C and E, are destroyed. Cooking is usually a combination of heat and water. Hot water dissolves more of the water soluble constituents such as sugar, vitamins, minerals, and amino acids. These are usually lost as the cooking water is often discarded.

On balance, cooking was probably beneficial during the "prechemical" stage of nutrition, for chemical additives were not available and thus could not react with food during the cooking process.

The Agricultural Era

About 10,000 years ago the introduction of herding and cropping secured a stable supply of large quantities of food and made man less dependent on gathering and hunting in the wild. There was no change in food technology except for storage. It was now possible to store grain for several years. Joseph advised the Pharaoh to store a seven-year supply of grain in preparation for the seven-year drought he predicted.

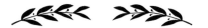

Agriculture forced a change in social habits, from a wandering, nomadic existence to the development of large cities. Territorial needs were changed from sparsely occupied areas with few interactions with others to huge, overcrowded, overconcentrated areas we know as modern cities.

Increasing food supply did not decrease our workload; likely the opposite came about. Agriculture is not an easy occupation. Farmers work hard and require a lot of food, probably much more than did the earlier gatherers and hunters. Did the story of Adam and Eve and their banishment into the real world signify the transition from hunting and gathering to agriculture? It has been estimated that hunters and gatherers were able to obtain enough food for their needs by working only two hours per day.

Primitive agriculture probably did not reduce the variety of food available; on the contrary, newer varieties of foods were probably selected and cropped. Modern agriculture has, of course, done the opposite because of its heavy reliance on single, high yielding varieties. Another consequence of agriculture was the increase of food for yeast. Man has domesticated yeast for production of alcoholic beverages and making bread. Or has the yeast species domesticated man to become a supplier of sugar and simple carbohydrates, both inside and outside of the body?

The Chemical Era

Agriculture provided a stable supply of meat and meat products and even more of cereals — barley, rice, wheat, corn, oats. It is impossible to visualize the huge populations on earth without this remarkable supply of food. Peoples have lived primarily on whole grain foods supplemented with small amounts of fish and meat. Cereals are easily grown, yield reliably, are easy to harvest, transport, and store. They retain the most important quality of foods — they are whole and alive. They can be ground, baked, cooked into a variety of foods, and sprouted. Of these

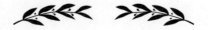

breads and cakes are the most important.

Ground grain has been used for making bread for thousands of years. These breads have ranged in quality from heavy whole grain bread to whiter, less heavy breads, but the technology for developing the pure white, fluffy, cottony, modern bread had not been invented. Grain could be ground, but only after the invention of the modern steel roller mill and accurate silk screens was it possible to separate wheat into coarse bran and germ, less coarse middlings, and the pure, fine, white flour, the endosperm, from which we make our white bread. Grinding and separating cereal components is the basis for much of our present food technology.

Grinding in itself was an important discovery since it made it possible to digest foods that could not be digested. Sifting out the most nutritious portion of the grain was not such a hot idea. But the wealthier classes enjoyed the whitest of flour and bread and this became the fashion. The poor people, slaves, and peasants had to be content with whole meal grain. They were of course lucky and must have been healthier than their masters and superiors. But even the whitest of flour was still not as white as is modern flour because the sieves which could screen out the bran and germ particles were discovered only about 300 years ago. Today the majority of people eat the poorest fraction of the wheat in their bread and pasta and feed the most nutritious parts to their animals.

Fermentation was also discovered several thousand years ago and was used to make alcoholic beverages. By the time the Old Testament was written wine was a staple of many diets and drunkenness was described. Pure sugar was unknown but honey was liked and harvested when it was located. The crystalization of sucrose from sugar cane juices became established about 300 years ago. Pure white sugar was very expensive during the rule of Queen Elizabeth. It was so expensive only the wealthy could afford to use it and

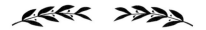

the average annual consumption in England was 5 pounds per person per year. The Queen was a sugar junky, and this probably rotted her teeth, making it essential for her to have iron plates. This could have accounted for her irritable personality later on in life. Today in England the consumption of all the sugars(sugar cane, sugar beet, and the syrups) runs close to 130 pounds per person per year. This is an average figure including infants. There is therefore 50 percent of the population who eat much more than that. The diet of some teenagers is 50 percent pure sugars.

As chemists became more skillful they discovered how to break foods down into its major components — the carbohydrates, fats, and proteins. Before vitamins and minerals were found to be as important as they are, it was believed by many nutritionists around 1900 that knowing the composition of foods in terms of these three major components was all that one needed to know since these three could be used to fashion a "perfect" diet. This notion was so popular in England that many of the children of the nobility died when they did not have wet nurses: many doctors thought that infant foods made only from starch, fat, and protein would be adequate to ensure good health.

By 1900 white bread and pure sugar had massively displaced whole grain cereals as food staples in high-tech societies. But since then there has been a major revolution in food technology. Dr. Ross Hume Hall in his book *Food for Naught: The Decline in Nutrition* estimates that since the Second World War consumption of overly processed food has increased from 25 percent of the total food intake to over 75 percent. This provides an estimate of the invasion of our food by chemistry.

Before I describe what chemistry has done to make our food less nutritious, if not harmful to our health, I should acknowledge the benefits. There are only three: food is cheaper; it can be stored for many years; and it requires less work to prepare for eating. The first advantage is, on close

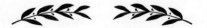

examination, seldom true. Today a pound of wheat costing under ten cents to the farmer, perhaps twenty five cents to the purchaser, will yield many more breakfasts than the same wheat converted into a cereal for over one dollar. The second advantage is real. Overly processed food can be stored much longer and it can be used to provide food when natural supplies are low. The detrimental effects of storage will be described further on. The main advantage is that less work is required. It is easier to buy bread than to bake it, easier to heat up a prepared meal. When both parents work this in an important advantage as there is no time to work full time in and outside the home. Convenience foods have made it easier for women to join the workforce.

Besides the nutritional disadvantages of cooking and refining foods, the modern high-tech diet is less nutritional because of chemical additives. Of the deleterious factors in overly processed foods the use of additives is among the worst. Additives are chemicals which are added in small quantities to impart special properties to the final food preparation. They are designed to impart taste, to preserve, to color, or to emulsify. The number of chemicals used for these purposes runs into the thousands. Governments allow them to be used on the basis that when tested on animals individually they appear to be non-lethal and non-toxic. But Dr. Hall has shown that toxicity tests of individual chemicals do not provide a true measure of the toxicity of a large number of chemicals present in food consumed for many years. An animal may survive one or two chemicals, but each additional one throws an additional burden on the body's defense systems. The body defends itself against chemicals by converting them to less toxic substances — by eliminating them in expired air, in urine, in feces, in sweat or by depositing them in skin and its appendages, hair and nails. The so-called theory of a toxic dose means that a dose below this level is non-toxic, that there is a "safe" level. This is no longer considered true for many compounds, and

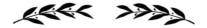

even when it is true, the safe level may be so narrow it is meaningless. Also the safe levels will depend on the presence of other additives which are negative factors and on nutrients which protect the body. Thus fiber and ascorbic acid protect animals against the toxic effect of cadmium. A diet deficient in fiber and low in ascorbic acid will thus enhance the toxic effect of additives. Another problem is that additives will combine with food under the influence of heat to form new, unnatural compounds. The toxicity of these has not been studied carefully.

Negative additives may be divided into two main groups: cosmetic additives and trace additives. Cosmetic additives include all the additives known to be present and permitted by law. They are used to alter taste, color, consistency, or stability and often include sugar as a bulk additive which is used because it perpetuates the addiction to sugar. These cosmetic additives do not enhance the nutritional quality of the food; on the contrary, they undoubtedly diminish it. I think we need a simple law which treats every processed food product as a drug. Before a drug can be released on prescription, it must be shown to be safe and effective for what is claimed it can do. If we applied the same idea to overly processed foods, we would have a much healthier society. Assume the product was the ubiquitous french fries. By this non-existent law, french fries would be fed to one group of growing animals, fresh potatoes to another. If the rate of growth on both sets of animals was identical, one could claim that commercial french fries are as nutritious as whole fresh, living potatoes. If animals on french fries grew half as fast, they would be labeled as having 50 percent of the nutritional quality of the original food. Each overly processed food would carry in the label this mark of quality as well as a list of the additives. This living test of food quality is the only way to measure the impact of processing on the product.

Trace additives are the additives which are not listed on the label because the manufacturer either does not know

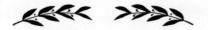

they are there or because there is no legal requirement that they be listed. Every organic chemist knows that it is impossible to synthesize an absolutely pure compound. One of the most expensive chemicals is pure water. Whenever any chemical is made, it contains traces of the other chemicals which were used in making it. Sugar is made from cane or beet and the final product is remarkably pure, perhaps 99.9 percent pure. Yet that 0.01 percent which is not sugar does contain traces of every chemical used in making it as well as traces of the natural products present in the original food. The same principle applies to every synthesized compound. Every chemical which enters any plant in the food production line, from the farmer to the store, is present in trace amounts somewhere in the food.

> **LAW**
>
> *I think we need a simple law which treats every processed food product as a drug. Before a drug can be released on prescription, it must be shown to be safe and effective for what is claimed it can do. If we applied the same idea to overly processed foods, we would have a much healthier society.*

A manufacturer who buys sugar to make a syrup or a pastry may know the product contains these traces and may not like it, but there is no requirement that it be listed or even detected. These trace additives are not added for any special reason. They are the contaminants from the process which converts natural food into overly processed food.

Toxicologists believe that these trace quantities are too low to be significant, but they have not proven this. If a person consumes 200 grams of sugar per day, he will also consume 0.02 grams (20 mg) of these contaminants per day. We have drugs that are highly active in these quantities; this amount of Haldol, a major tranquilizer, would keep most people totally incapacitated, and one-tenth of one milligram of LSD will incapacitate most normal people for up to one day. We know Haldol and LSD are not present in sugar, but the principle remains — we must not assume

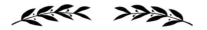

these small quantities are inactive.

We can minimize the amount of trace additives in our food by avoiding overly processed foods whenever it is possible and by using processed foods which have undergone the least amount of processing. Thus rolled oats is nearly as good as whole oats and is much healthier than any sugared cereal with an oat base.

There is also a class of additives that can be said to be helpful. The added substances enhance the nutritional quality of the final product. These positive additives are primarily nutrients, such as minerals and vitamins. Thus enriched white flour is better than ordinary white flour but is not as nutritious as whole wheat flour. The use of nutrient additives allows companies to make claims for the nutritional value of their products which are dubious, if not false.

DEAD, STALE, TOXIC . . .

Another way to understand the differences between a "primitive" or pure diet and a modern or high-tech diet is to compare them using this table:

PRIMITIVE	HIGH-TECH
Whole	Artifact
Alive	Dead
Fresh	Stale
Varied	Monotonous
Non-Toxic	Toxic
Scarce	Abundant
Endogenous	Exogenous
Natural Flavor	Synthetic
Simple	Complex

Artifact

Much modern high-tech food is *artifact*. By this I mean that foods are broken down to their constituent fractions, such

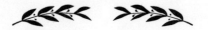

as starch, sugars, fats, oils, and protein, and these are then recombined to make preparations which have the appearance of natural food but are not. For example, it is possible to buy tomato soup which contains no tomatoes but in appearance and flavor would lead one to believe that it is really tomato soup. It is possible to buy overly processed cheese which has little of the original cheese in it, and overly processed fish or crab which appears to be crab. Only the bad odor before it is fried will give it away. It is possible to buy overly processed turkey which is turkey protein pressed out to look like slices of real turkey meat but isn't. These artifacts are dangerous because they are made to look and to taste like food. The average person eating these foods would naturally assume that they are what they appear to be and yet they would not contain the nutrient quality that was present in the original food. Overly processed foods not only fool the senses of taste and smell, but they also make it impossible to judge the quality of the food by using the subterfuge of appearing to be real food. Artifacts are pseudo foods, preparations which are made up from a combination of artifacts or fractions of the original foods.

Dead

Much modern high-tech food is *dead*. Alive food does not store well. Animal products very quickly deteriorate due to oxidation, enzymatic activity, and decomposition by bacteria and fungi. These changes can be inhibited by using freezing, by drying, or by cooking the products. Cooking will slow down the rate of decomposition. The food is also preserved by the addition of chemicals which retard the growth of bacteria and fungi and which are antioxidants, thus retarding the oxidation of the food. Milk can be heat treated at such a high temperature that it is stable even at room temperature for a long time. It does not turn sour because the lactobacilli which ought to be present to sour the milk are destroyed. Modern bread has many chemicals

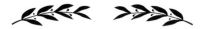

in it which prevent it from aging and turning hard. Bread without these additives will be fresh one day and will be stale the second day. One of the main additives used to improve the baking quality and cosmetic properties of white bread, potassium bromate, is being disallowed in Canada. Canned foods can be stored for years as can frozen foods. The least damaging way of storing food is to freeze it, followed by canning. Removing the enzymes and the reducing compounds will decrease the rate at which these foods oxidize. Removing vitamins and minerals will discourage bacteria and fungi, which must also have these nutrients to grow. The more a food is deprived of its easily lost and destroyed nutrients the more apt is that food to be stable. This is why starch extracted from wheat or potatoes is much more stable and can be stored much longer than the original plant material. But the price for the increase in stability is an equal decrease in the nutritive quality of those products. The price, however, is paid by the consumer, not by the high-tech industry which creates these long-lived stable foods. One of the aims of processing good food like wheat or oats is to convert them to a final product which costs a lot more, is much more stable, tastes sweet — and is much more dangerous to our health. We increase the value of products by converting good food into junk. In economic terms this is value-added.

Stale

Stale is another quality of high-tech food. Most of what I have said about dead applies as well to this term. As a rule overly processed food is both dead and stale.

Monotonous

The term monotonous refers to the limited variety of foods which are available. This will be surprising to shoppers who have not thought about it, especially when they are cruising around a supermarket with 15,000 to 20,000 different items

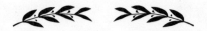

on the shelves. They must think that we have an enormous variety of foods. If the prepared breakfast section carries 50 different products, are we in fact having access to 50 different foods. We are not because they are all artifacts made from oats, wheat, rice, sugar, flavors, and other additives packaged in attractive boxes. Even if we eat a wide variety from each of the 50 items, we are still eating the same three grains and sugar.

We increase the value of products by converting good food into junk. In economic terms this is value-added.

A monotonous diet is responsible for many of the health problems present in high-tech societies. There are two reasons for this. First, there will be a shortage of vitamins, minerals, and essential fatty acids. A diet which contains a variety of cereals, vegetables, fruit, and animal products is much more apt, even if only because of chance, to provide an adequate amount of these essential nutrients. For over 99 percent of man's existence on earth, there was no need to apply intelligence towards food selection. The only important fact was whether the food was poisonous or not. Among the foods found not to be poisonous, it was good enough to eat everything else provided there was an amply variety available. Since there was no abundance of any one food, it was necessary to eat what was available from all the foods. Thus primitive tribes living as hunters-gatherers would eat everything in their path that was edible. The variety depended on what was available in their community and varied from morning to night, from week to week, from season to season. Variety, combined with the absence of high-tech food products, was adequate to maintain a reasonable state of health. Studies of the natives of the Kalihari desert showed that they were healthy. However, these peoples have been forced into villages, their life style has been altered, and they have been introduced to the limited monotonous high-tech diet. There has been a remarkable deterioration in their health. We will

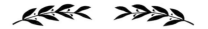

also see this problem develop in a new tribe of people "found" in Papua New Guinea, the Liawep tribe. There are 79 members in the tribe, the Toronto *Globe and Mail* reported in a 1993 article. They had never before had contact with our world but have already been exposed to tea, salt, and sugar since being found. There is no doubt that they will take to these like children to candy and that their health will deteriorate in a remarkable manner over the next 20 years. This is the first introduction of the high-tech diet to a primitive people still living on the original natural diet to which they had adapted.

We have seen the same phenomenon closer to home. About 50 years ago the average grocery store contained few items, often in bulk, chiefly vegetables, grains, and fruit. A person ignorant of nutrition could by chance purchase what would be needed to sustain good health. Suppose one were instructed to purchase 12 different items. The number of good items would be greater than the number of poor items nutritionally. That person could be healthy using those 12 items that had been selected at random, without any intellectual knowledge of which foods should be eaten or not. This is no longer possible in the modern supermarket. Out of the 15,000 items available about 50 would be suitable to maintain health. The vast majority of items would not be nourishing since they are the product of the high-tech industry. About the only safe place in which to shop is around the walls, for that is where the vegetables and fruits, the meat and fish, the dairy products, much of the frozen goods, and the breads are found.

Recently, I read a report that food processing companies were becoming concerned about the number of people who only shop around the walls, thereby avoiding most of their products. They were trying to work out a way to entice shoppers to go to the center of the store. Perhaps one day they will mix the processed foods with the foods naturally available around the walls so that people will be forced to at least

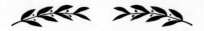

look at these products. If one were to instruct a robot to select at random 12 items from the store, very few items would provide any nourishment. The major part of that shopping expedition would consist of junk — and a person living on the diet could not remain well. A combination of variety and good food is all that is needed for us to remain well. Our appetite will ensure that we eat a variety of food, for we tend to become satiated with too much of one food at one time. The body seems to have an instinctive revulsion at eating too much of anything unless, of course, that food had been corrupted by the addition of sugar, salt, and other additives so commonly used. It was easier for the naive shopper to buy food that would maintain health 50 years ago than it is today.

The second reason for the ill-effects of a monotonous diet is that the probability of developing allergic reactions to foods is directly related to the proportion of our diet occupied by that food. That is why most of the allergic reactions are to foods which are staples for that region. In England tea allergies are more common than they are in the U.S.A. In countries where rice is the main staple, there will be more allergic reactions to rice. In wheat countries, wheat products will be common allergens, and in countries where corn is used extensively and corn by-products are incorporated into prepared foods, corn allergy will be common. In my practice I have estimated that between 25 and 40 percent of patients have one or another type of dairy product allergy.

Allergic reactions to food can become evident at any time in life. Infants fed on formula (milk and sugar) often become allergic to both milk and sugar. They then may have symptoms like colic, frequent colds, runny noses, rashes, itches, and so on. Later these somatic symptoms may subside only to be replaced by behavioral changes and learning disorders. Many hyperactive and learning disordered children have dairy allergies. Wetting the bed is a very common milk allergy. Later in life, by the time they are adult, they may have

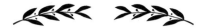

developed an aversion to milk but be excessively fond of cheese. Young people with a violent nature and who are often in trouble with the law have been found to eat excessive amounts of sugar and milk products. They are often very immature in their behavior; I have considered them as infants who have not yet been weaned from their milk. One such individual had for breakfast each morning a quart of Coca Cola and a quart of milk. Another middle-aged man, who had been in prison several years for assaulting a police officer, carried a quart bottle of concentrated sugar with him all the time. When he became tired, he would drink that solution. This indicates a food allergy is present. One of the treatments for food allergy is to rotate the diet, which means introducing variation into the diet. The illnesses and diseases caused by milk allergies and milk-sugar combinations will be discussed fully later in the book.

Toxic

Modern high-tech foods are often *toxic*. By toxic I do not mean they contain poisons which will kill rapidly, but taken over long periods of time, years and decades, they produce a state of chronic ill health. Before additives can be incorporated into foods they have to pass certain toxicity tests. The test may simply be one where the additive has been used for a long time and has apparently not made anyone ill. The modern test is to add the chemicals to the diet of animals and to determine the toxic dose, the so-called LD_{50}. This is the amount which will kill half the animals given the chemical over a period of time. The chemicals are also tested to determine whether they have any effect on the growth of young animals and whether they interfere with pregnancy or the development of the fetus. These are usually short term experiments. They are seldom given to animals over a major fraction of their lives, so they do not accurately test the effect of chronic use. A second objection

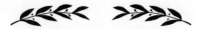

is that additives are tested singly. When given in combinations, the toxic properties of these chemicals can be additive and probably are. Most high-tech foods contain more than two additives. Seldom is the exact mixture of the food used in tests to determine its long term effect. The third objection to testing is that the additives are tested on animals who are fed properly. Laboratory animals are given nutritious food of the type they have adapted to. A healthy animal is better able to resist the toxic effects of chemicals. However, the diet for most people is inadequate and they are less able to cope with the chemicals present in their food. The major additive is sugar, followed by salt, but each person also consumes 5 pounds of other chemicals each year in their food. The diseases caused by overconsumption of sugar and salt will be described further on.

Abundant

Modern diets are *abundant,* more accurately, they are *excessive.* Before high-tech foods became available, the common problem facing mankind was starvation. We had adapted to this problem by developing mechanisms for storing extra calories which could be drawn on during these periods of inadequate food supply. It is much like the camel's ability to store water to be used when none is available. Usually what food was available was of pretty good quality. There simply was not enough. Today there is no starvation in high-tech societies, unless it is created by war and other man-made activities. There are many people who believe they are not getting enough food, but the proportion of our population which is too thin, which suffers from protein-calorie deficiency, from marasmus, is very small. On the contrary, perhaps 25 percent of the population is overweight, even among people seeking extra food from community agencies. The problem in modern times is that there are too many calories but that the foods which carry these calories are lacking in nutritional quality. They are

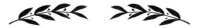

short of vitamins, minerals, and fiber — excessive in sugars, fat, and oils. The diseases generated by the over consumption of high-tech food will be described further on when I deal with the Saccharine Disease.

Exogenous

Our modern diet is *exogenous.* This refers to foods which are gathered, grown, or raised in areas of the world which are climactically much different. An example would be the consumption of fruit native to the tropics in cold countries like Sweden or Canada, or the importation of apples grown in Canada to the tropics. The essential fatty acid composition of these exotic foods will differ significantly from the composition of the vegetables and fruits raised in the same areas. Cold climate animals and vegetables contain a higher proportion of unsaturated fatty acids relative to the saturated fatty acid. The essential fatty acids make living organisms more cold tolerant.

Artificially Flavored

High-tech processed food is *artificially flavored.* Chemical flavor additives have no value in nutrition except for cosmetic purposes and over the long haul will be found to be toxic. More and more additives are being removed from the market, usually after many complaints, after some testing, by government decree. Flavor additives also destroy the ability of our senses to distinguish good from bad food, and in this way add to the general burden of ill health caused by these high-tech diets. The major flavoring substance is sugar, followed by salt.

Complex

The last adjective we can apply to the modern high-tech diet is *complex.* High-tech foods are composed of a large number of items. For example, one breakfast cereal lists the following ingredients: "whole oat flour, degermed yellow

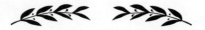

corn meal, wheat starch, sugar, salt, dextrose, vitamins, reduced iron, calcium carbonate, color, trisodium phosphate." This is one of the better cereals, containing less than a gram of sugar per serving. There is a reason for each ingredient. The major item is the oats. Degermed corn is used since germ would make the this product more unstable and it could not be stored as long. The sugar, salt, and dextrose (another sugar) are flavoring agents. Color is added with phosphate to stabilize the color. The vitamins and iron enhance its nutritional quality and try to restore what has been lost in the processing.

The main problem with complex foods is that the consumer does not know what is present in the food. It may contain ingredients to which we are allergic. Many patients have a multiple allergy syndrome and are reactive to almost every chemical. The presence of so many chemicals increases the likelihood that they will have an additive effect in causing toxicity and ill health. The foods we have adapted to contain a combination of nutrients which can be dealt with by our digestive apparatus. If we were given the 50 or so pure nutrients and asked to provide the proper balance for all our needs, there would be great difficulty. The combinations of ingredients placed in these complex foods has not been worked out by nutritional tests. They have been worked out on the basis of economics, cosmetic properties(taste and smell and appearance), and the need to prepare mixtures which will not deteriorate in time.

It is claimed that the complexity of the label should not be a deterrent since a label on natural food would be even more complex if every ingredient were listed. The difference is that in whole natural food none of the ingredients are in a pure state. They are all part of a very complex series of molecules. And they have been around for so long that the body is accustomed to them and knows how to deal with them. They are "orthomolecular" products. The synthetics added to food are xenobiotic or foreign and therefore they present major problems to the body.

DIETARY
DISEASES

❧

Over 75 percent of our current diet consists of processed food. This diet is deficient in fiber, too rich in processed fats, too rich in simple sugars, and deficient in vitamins, minerals, and essential fatty acids, the omega-3 type. It is also too rich in additives. The average person consumes about 140 pounds of additives per year. Of this, 102 pounds is sucrose, 13 pounds is dextrose, 15 pounds salt, 8 pounds pepper, mustard, baking soda, citric acid, and 26 other common kitchen substances, and 2.1 pounds comes from 2400 synthetic cosmetic additives. Trace additives coming from processed products used to make food mixtures are not included.

This unnatural diet is responsible for the large number of sick people today. When they give up this diet for a natural orthomolecular diet, the majority of patients become well. When they revert back to the high-tech diet, they again become ill. I have seen this effect on thousands of my patients over the past 40 years, as have other orthomolecular physicians.

> *Over 75 percent of our current diet consists of processed food. This diet is deficient in fiber, too rich in processed fats, too rich in simple sugars, and deficient in vitamins, minerals, and essential fatty acids, the omega-3 type.* **LAW**

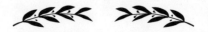

The diseases caused by the modern unnatural diet may be classified into a few simple causal groups. Although there is one major disease caused by malnutrition, so many different organ systems are involved that it is simpler to follow the common medical pattern of describing individual diseases such as peptic ulcer, gall bladder disease, and hypoglycemia. But it is important to remember that these are all diseases caused by inadequacies of the diet and that therefore the treatment for each one of these diseases will be almost the same — restore the natural diet and thus the adaptation. A logical way to relate the inadequacies of the diet with the various diseases is to work with the compositional changes in the food supply due to high-tech processing. The modern diet is a low fiber, high sugar, high fat, high additive, high calorie diet, which at the same time is deficient in micronutrients such as vitamins and minerals. I will describe how each of these factors plays a role in making people sick and the kind of diseases suffered as a result.

LOW FIBER

Fiber is mainly carbohydrates. It is the portion of the vegetable and animal material that remains in the gastrointestinal system because it cannot be completely digested. There is much more fiber in plant food than in animal food. Plant fiber can be divided into three different types: the cereal fibers, the vegetable fibers, and the fruit fibers. Foods which are low in fibrous materials do not leave enough residue in the bowel, resulting in very small stools which tend to be hard and infrequent.

People living on a diet low in fiber-rich foods tend to have many diseases which were not present in people who consume whole foods which are rich in fiber. Constipation is the hallmark of the low fiber diet. Dr. Burkett has observed that in nations there was an inverse relationship between the size of the stools and the size of the hospitals. With small

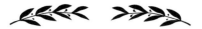

stools he found that large hospitals were needed. After spending many years traveling and lecturing about his findings, the idea took hold that high fiber foods were better. Western medicine is so accustomed to working with fractions of foods, however, that it ignored his finding that the fiber was needed as a constituent of whole foods and they began to study the use of fiber by itself in the form of bran or pure fibers. They soon found that the pure fibers by themselves were not nearly as helpful as the whole foods. Fiber is very important but primarily as a component of whole foods. Bran and other high fiber foods are useful in many circumstances, but they should not be used to replace the whole foods rich in fiber.

All whole foods are rich in fiber compared to overly processed foods; a person consuming whole foods need not worry very much about adding additional fiber to the diet. A person living primarily on overly processed foods will probably have a major deficiency of fiber and will suffer the consequences. These are constipation or diarrhea alternating with constipation. I define constipation as movements which occur less frequently than one per day with stools which are hard, small in volume, and require much effort to expel. Ideally one should have one to two movements per day with large bulky stools which are semi-fluid and which are expelled with minimal effort. Diarrhea is present when the stools are very watery and very frequent.

Normally the contractions and relaxations of the small and large bowel propel the food towards the large colon and rectum from where it is expelled. But it is difficult for the bowel to propel the food onward if there is little material to grab on to. Low fiber foods are so thoroughly digested in the stomach and in the small intestine that when the contents reach the colon there is little fiber present. As the bowel contents travel onward, nutrients released by the digestion and water are absorbed. At the same time the bacteria and fungi present in the colon become more active. By the time the

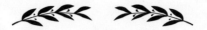

feces is expelled, its bulk may consist entirely of the dead bodies of yeast, bacteria, and other organisms which have converted the fiber to other insoluble material.

A low fiber diet can also lead to colitis, diverticulosis, hemorrhoids, gall bladder disease, appendicitis, and cancer of the colon. The combination of too much sugar and too little fiber is a factor in causing hypercholesterolemia and atherosclerosis. Coronary disease is one outcome, as is stroke. There is little doubt that if we reverted back to a high fiber, low sugar diet, coronary disease would almost disappear and heart surgeons would have little to do. The lack of vitamin C is another main factor in causing hardening of the arteries but other vitamins such as niacin and pyridoxine also are involved as are other nutrients. The low fiber, high sugar diet is low in many essential nutrients, including these vitamins.

> **LAW**
>
> *There is little doubt that if we reverted back to a high fiber, low sugar diet, coronary disease would almost disappear and heart surgeons would have little to do.*

HIGH SUGAR

Two common sugars circulate in the blood; glucose, which is very essential and safe when the concentration is not too high, and fructose, which is not safe. All carbohydrates are broken down or hydrolyzed during digestion into the simple sugars. The simple monosaccharides are then absorbed through the intestinal wall and enter the bloodstream. This sugar provides energy for all the cells of the body. If the concentration of glucose in the blood drops too far, cells become starved for food energy, and the brain may suffer enough deficiency that the person will faint and go into a coma. This is what happens when a diabetic takes too much insulin. This drives the blood sugar too far down by increasing the amount of glucose which the cells take up. Glucose released by digestion and absorbed into the blood will not

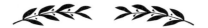

cause any harm if the food being digested is the whole food, such as whole wheat, carrots, brown rice, and so on. The rate of entry into the blood is slow, controlled, and accompanied by the nutrients in the whole grain. Each molecule of sugar released in this way comes with a package of other nutrients, vitamins, and minerals, and these are available to the body for the processing of the sugar molecules into energy and into other products.

In sharp contrast are the so-called free sugars which have already been refined, liberated from every nutritional component of the foods in which they were made. They can be eaten very quickly so that in addition to the quantities consumed, which are excessive, they are absorbed too rapidly. This throws an enormous burden on the body which has to deal with all the sugar.

Whole foods contain very little free sugar. Even ripe fruit will contain less than 20 percent sugar, and fruits which have not been altered by plant breeders contain even less. Natural fruit tends to be less sweet, but plant breeders have selected for sweetness since this appeals to the taste of the public. The major source of sugar before the advent of the chemical age was the honey that our ancestors gathered. With the development of cane and beets as good sources of sugar, it became possible to consume huge amounts of free sugars. This has had a major impact on the health of the populations which follow the high-tech diet.

The combination of low fiber and high sugar in the diet creates the condition called the Saccharine Disease. The symptoms are peptic ulcer due to a deficiency of protein when gastric juice is secreted while eating. Drinking a sugared, carbonated drink stimulates secretion of acid which finds no protein to which it can be attached. The excess of calories, sugar, other simple carbohydrates, fat, and lack of

---

The combination of low fiber and high sugar in the diet creates the condition called the Saccharine Disease. **LAW**

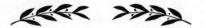

exercise are factors in causing obesity and diabetes mellitus, especially the late maturity or adult onset type. It is probably more accurate to consider this type of diabetes a variant of hypoglycemia. Relative hypoglycemia afflicts nearly two-thirds of all psychiatric populations and 100 percent of all addict populations. Out of several hundred tests, I have yet to find one alcoholic with a normal five-hour glucose tolerance curve.

Excess sugar also provides a medium for yeast which inhabits our gastro-intestinal tract. The combination of too much sugar, antibiotics which destroy normal bacterial flora and allow yeast overgrowth, and birth control medication which encourages vaginal overgrowth of yeast is largely responsible for yeast infection that troubles so many people. In addition, chemotherapy or steroid therapy decreases the immune defense system. A combination of yeast overgrowth and decreased immune defense may be responsible for a number of auto immune diseases, such as multiple sclerosis, perhaps lupus, muscular dystrophies, rheumatoid arthritis, and so on.

The effect of high sugar, low fiber on gastrointestinal (g.i.) physiology is becoming clearer. When only whole foods are consumed, the masticated food, the enzymes and fluid added to it, and the products of enzymatic digestion are propelled through the g.i. tract, clearing the system in less than 24 hours. The longer the food remains in the gut, the higher is the bacterial and yeast cell count, for these organisms thrive in a warm, wet medium containing partially digested food. There normally is a gradient of bacterial count which is lowest in the duodenum and highest in the colon. The whole g.i. tract functions to keep bacterial yeast count low in the small intestine where most of the nutrients are absorbed, while allowing bacterial count to rise in the colon where there is little absorption. The products of bacterial metabolism, which are harmful, are thus retained in the colon and excreted with the feces. But the longer the food is stored the

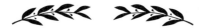

greater the contamination. The food in the stomach is sterilized by the strong hydrochloric acid in the stomach. Once food starts traveling down the small intestines, bacterial count slowly goes up. But peristalsis or the successive wave-like contractions of the g.i. system keeps feeding lightly contaminated material into more heavily contaminated material. The passage of food tends to decrease invasion by bacteria of the intestine. Reverse peristalsis would throw highly contaminated material to an area where it is usually not present. In the absence of sufficient fiber, peristalsis is decreased, leaving food in the intestinal system much longer. As a result bacterial content of the feces is much higher in areas of the intestine where this normally does not occur.

The small intestine must be kept bacteria free. When too much sugar is present, it stimulates overgrowth of yeast. The saccharine inducing diet also leads to bacterial and yeast overgrowth in areas of the intestine where this should not occur. Fasting, with or without enemas, has been used for many decades to treat a variety of diseases, ranging from cancer and arthritis to serious psychiatric problems. Perhaps the common factor is the elimination or marked reduction of candida or yeast infection from the gastrointestinal tract. A four day fast (96 hour) would eliminate yeast from most people. But for a person with a fast transit time, one or two days might be enough. A water diet would be more therapeutic than a juice diet, because the sugar in the juice would provide nourishment for the yeast. A combination of enema and fasting would be more effective than a simple fast, especially for people with sluggish bowels.

HIGH FAT

Life would be impossible on a diet with no fat. Hardly any food is totally devoid of fat. It is an essential constituent. In natural food it is present in an intricate complex mixture of protein and carbohydrates with their essential vitamins,

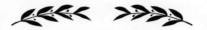

minerals, and enzymes. There are very few natural foods which contain too much fat. If everyone followed the principles of the natural diet, there would be no need to be concerned about getting too much fat. But the free availability of fats and oils creates a major problem and most people consume too much fat. The North American diet contains about 40 percent fat, whereas the optimum amount of fat expressed as calories probably varies between 10 and 20 percent depending on the climate.

Fat provides much more energy per gram, 9 calories, than sugar and protein which provides about 4 calories. It is thus an important source of energy, and in animals fat is the main storage depot for calories. When the consumption is greater than the use of energy, the extra energy is stored in the body in the fat depots. You will know where they are by looking at any person, especially when they are overweight or obese. The ability to store excess calories was a marvelous device for balancing out the food intake and expenditure. During famine or milder food shortages, our ancestors would draw upon the fat which they had accumulated during periods when they were able to consume too much. Nature also provided for nourishing fetuses and babies by providing women with more storage capacity for calories which would be drawn upon during pregnancy and lactation. If we had to depend upon carbohydrates to store our energy, we would be over 200 percent as bulky. Movement would be impossible.

Too little fat is undesirable, for it will be impossible or very difficult to maintain weight, to have enough energy for physical activity, to fight cold weather, to absorb fat soluble vitamins, and to provide the essential fatty acids. On a low fat diet people will be hungry and this will tempt many to increase their intake of sugars in order to replace the missed calories. But our major problem today in high-tech societies is too much fat, not too little. That is because fat artifacts are so readily available. Butter, milk, cream, cheeses, margarine,

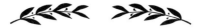

and liquid oils are staple items used in cooking. The favorite companion is sugar. Sweets consist of a mixture of sugar and fat. The sweet taste and the composition of the fat makes this a very attractive food item. The doughnut represents the acme of the high-tech diet, for it consists of white flour, sugar, and fat.

Too much fat is much more pathological since it causes obesity and all the complications that go along with it. We are now in the midst of the high fat, high cholesterol paradigm, and it will take many years to overcome this, as many years as it took to become the common diet. However, the role of fat in causing cardiovascular disease, coronary occlusion, and strokes has been exaggerated. I believe that too much sucrose and other sugars is much more important as a cause of arteriosclerosis and that this factor has been almost totally ignored. The usual advice given to patients who want to know how to decrease the chance of getting heart disease is to exercise, stop smoking, learn to relax, and decrease their intake of fat. This is very sound advice and everyone should follow it, but it probably won't decrease the incidence of heart disease, unless other measures are also adopted such as reducing the sugar intake. Dr. I. Shine studied the incidence of heart disease on the island of St. Helena. On this island in the South Atlantic Ocean, 1200 miles west of Africa, the natives already follow all these basic four prescriptions. The land is hilly and there are no cars so they have to walk a lot. Very few smoke. They are relaxed and their fat intake is fairly low. Still, they have a very high incidence of heart disease. But their intake of sugar since 1900 has increased to the level in England and in Canada, about 125 pounds per person per year.

The processed diet of modern technological societies contains too much fat and its quality has been deteriorated

The processed diet of modern technological societies contains too much fat and its quality has been deteriorated by the processing.

LAW

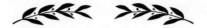

by the processing. Whole foods are seldom very rich in fat and what is present is not destroyed by heat or by oxidation. Not many whole foods contain as much as 20 percent fat. But when the fats are separated from the food, it becomes possible to consume very large quantities. These processed fats include butter, cream, margarine, and all the oils. The problem with butter and cream is that it is too easy to eat large quantities and so overload the body with calories. The problem with commercial oils and margarines is they are heat treated and oxidized. The natural fatty acids are changed by heat into unnatural fatty acids. This creates problems for the body, hastening atherosclerosis; another consequence is the destruction of essential fatty acids (EFAs). These fatty acids are highly reactive and easily become rancid when stored and therefore must be removed. This deprives us of EFAs which creates a variety of pathological conditions. There is also a displacement of fat-rich foods rich in EFAs by sources which contain very little. Crops which grow in warm areas do not need protection against cold and therefore have little unsaturated fatty acids. Temperate crops, such as wheat, oats, and flax, require more; unsaturated fatty acids have lower melting points. Flax and its oil, linseed oil, were used as staples many years ago. They have been replaced by corn, coconut, canola, and other warmer crop oils. As a result we consume only 20 percent of the EFAs consumed before 1950.

There is no doubt that fats are involved in atherosclerosis, that high blood cholesterol and high blood triglycerides increase the risk of developing atherosclerosis. I also believe that there is no relationship between consumption of whole foods and atherosclerosis. These foods will prevent elevation of blood fats, except in familial hypercholesterolemia. But I would expect that consumption of pure fats is related. Thus there should be no fear of eating eggs, a whole food, but I would be concerned over utilization of butter, margarine, and the commercial oils. If epidemiologists would report total fat intake, fat intake from whole foods, and fat intake

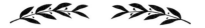

from butter, cream, margarine, and oils they would have a much clearer view of the relationship of fats to atherosclerosis, coronary disease, and strokes.

VITAMIN AND MINERAL DEFICIENCIES

Although the classic deficiency diseases are not necessarily produced by the modern high-tech diet, for we rarely see scurvy, beri beri, pellagra, or rickets, this diet does cause modern deficiency diseases with vague, diffuse symptoms. These patients share in common the fact that usual clinical examination and laboratory tests do not reveal a cause for their fatigue, distress, and malaise. Most are eventually labeled as psychosomatic or psychiatric. For this reason, it is more appropriate to call them sub-clinical deficiencies. Medical literature contains reports of sub-clinical deficiencies, especially among residents of hospitals and nursing homes. These deficiencies and dependencies will be discussed in great detail later.

EXCESSIVE ADDITIVES

We are just becoming aware of the impact additives have on health. It is my impression they are a factor in diminishing the immune defenses. They also play a role in causing learning and behavioral disorders in some children.

In July 1991 many scientists met at the Wingspread Conference Center, Racine, Wisconsin to consider the effect of chemicals dumped into the environment on development. Their consensus statement concluded "a large number of man-made chemicals that have been released into the environment, as well as a few natural ones, have the potential to disrupt the endocrine system of animals, including humans." Four general points were made: (1) the chemicals may have entirely different effects on the embryo, fetus, or perinatal organisms than on the adult; (2) the effects are most often

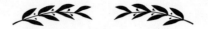

manifested in offspring, not in the exposed parent; (3) the timing of exposure in the developing organism is crucial; (4) although critical exposure occurs during embryonic development, obvious manifestations may not occur until maturity. They warned that "some of the developmental impairments reported in humans today are seen in adult offspring of parents exposed to synthetic hormone disrupters . . . released in the environment." Some of the xenobiotics, like the PCBs and dioxins, are of particular concern because they persist in the environment and bioaccumulate in the food chain. Most of our food has been treated with pesticides, designed to kill organisms, but has not been tested for endocrine and multigeneration effects.

Another example is phosphates present in many of our processed foods, especially in the soft drinks. For some sensitive children this is a major cause of hyperactivity. The soft, astringent drinks so very popular are loaded with several of the most causal factors in hyperactivity — sugar, phosphates, and a variety of chemicals including dyes.

The majority of cases of cancer are due to environmental factors — chiefly the chemical pollutants in our air, water, soil, and food. But inasmuch as most of us do not develop cancer, there must be a second set of factors, the immune defenses. Our modern processed foods with all the defects, especially with the additives present, must play a role in decreasing immune resistance. It has been shown, for example, that leukocytes deficient in ascorbic acid are not able to engulf bacteria. Furthermore, the only substance known to increase interferon production in the body is ascorbic acid, often deficient in the high-tech diet.

Auto-immune diseases (the immune system attacks normal tissues) include diseases such as rheumatoid arthritis, multiple sclerosis, lupus, perhaps muscular dystrophy. Treatment for these conditions is largely palliative using steroid hormones and immunosuppresents. When they do help, improvement is temporary and partial. Dr. O. Truss

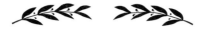

has suggested that chronic yeast (candida) infection may lead to an immobilization of the natural defense system and a distortion of the relationship between various types of leukocytes. Anti-yeast treatment allowed these defenses to be restored. The main treatment was the anti-fungal drug mycostatin.

Modern high-tech food additives have the same impact on children who experience learning and behavioral (hyperactivity) disorders and on adolescents who exhibit antisocial and later criminal behavior. I have seen how addiction to sugar has paved the way to violent behavior in adolescents and adults. These addicted children invariably begin to steal money from their parents, later from others in order to buy sweets. They may not be caught for a long time, for parents find it difficult to believe their children will do this. They may be caught only occasionally. If they are punished 10 percent of the time, this is a small price to pay for having gotten the desired sugar. Once the pattern has been established it will continue into adolescence where the wants are different but the method of achieving them the same. Now they steal for drugs, for alcohol, for cigarettes until the criminal pattern of behavior is well established.

> *Modern high-tech food additives have the same impact on children who experience learning and behavioral (hyperactivity) disorders and on adolescents who exhibit antisocial and later criminal behavior.*   **LAW**

The New York Public School System (803 schools) introduced a diet policy which lowered sucrose, synthetic food colors, and two preservatives over four years. This was followed by a 15.7 percent increase in mean academic percentile rating above the rest of the nation's schools that used the same tests. It has also been shown that behavioral problems decreased 48 percent in a detention facility involving 276 delinquents during the year the diet was changed. Many other institutions discovered the same facts.

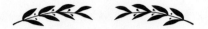

Decreasing sugar and additives lowered the incidence of bad behavior. Anyone who doubts this need only see what happens when their children are placed upon a sugar free diet for at least two weeks. It is important to do this before advising children to avoid sweets permanently and totally.

Additives may also cause mood disorders. The symptoms include fatigue, depression, and anxiety, in various mixes. Most sufferers of the very severe and manic depressions do not fall into this category but there is evidence that they are suffering from severe allergic reactions, perhaps to foods. I have seen many patients with mood disorders recover when the proper nutritional and supplements were used.

The relationship of the schizophrenias to nutrition is not as clear. But since the most effective treatments include modification of the diet and the use of vitamin B-3 and vitamin B-6 as the main supplements, it must be a major factor. There are patients who are allergic to foods as well as to other chemicals. I have treated over 100 patients who had not responded well enough to my program of drugs and vitamins by having them do a four day fast. The majority were well by the fifth day. When the food they were allergic too was re-introduced, they promptly became psychotic again.

COMBINED DISEASES

Now that we have seen the diseases caused by the modern high-tech diet — low fiber, high sugar, high fat, vitamin and mineral deficient, excessive additives — we can look at the combined affects of these unnatural dietary practices on the digestive system. To do this systematically I will begin from the mouth and teeth and follow the gastrointestinal (g.i.) tract to the anus. This is a one organ system and not a series of individual and separate organs. If the mouth is sick, so is the rest of the g.i. tract.

The modern diet causes dental caries. Deposits of sugar from the food are not properly swept away from the teeth

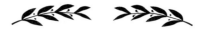

by the food and by the saliva because of an excess of sugar and a deficiency of fiber. Foods rich in fiber must be chewed and in this process the teeth are cleaned.

The loss of the sense of taste and smell due to mineral deficiency is a minor problem in young people but becomes more and more important in elderly people. It is caused by a deficiency of zinc and perhaps by an accumulation of copper. There is nothing which destroys appetite as fast as a distorted sense of taste and smell. Foods become tasteless or bitter or flat. It may be possible to recognize what the food is but the taste becomes so objectionable that the patient cannot eat and may become very depressed. A rapid test of the sense of taste can be conducted by administering a solution of zinc sulfate. Normal people find this solution very sharp and bitter and objectionable. But when they have lost their sense of taste due to a deficiency of zinc, they will not find any unusual taste in this solution. A blood test for zinc and copper will help establish the diagnosis. I was sent an elderly woman who was very depressed because she could no longer taste her food. She had seen over ten different doctors in order to get help but nothing they could do was effective. I started her on tablets of zinc sulfate which she took for over two years without any improvement. Then I started her on zinc sulfate solution giving her 100 mg of zinc per day. Within a few months she began to recover and she has been well for about five years. Her sense of taste is not fully normal but has improved so much she can enjoy her food and she is not depressed.

Patients who suffer from eating disorders such as obesity or bulimia probably have an abnormal appetite for carbohydrates and sweets for a reason which has not been considered and which has to do with the need to obtain enough of the essential nutrients. In 1949 an investigator ran a very interesting experiment with rats. These rats were kept in a running cage, a device which allowed the rats to run and which would measure the distance run during any

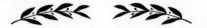

one day. Normal rats fed a good healthy rat diet would run a certain number of miles each day, around three or so. When the same animals were given a diet low in calories, they would double the amount that they ran. This is understandable since in nature it is hunger which motivates animals to wake up and start hunting. A lion after a feed will sleep for many hours until aroused once more by hunger. This is a life saving reflex probably present in all animals. When the same rats were given a diet that had enough calories but was deficient in the B vitamins, they ran as much as the fasting rats, even though they were not starving. My explanation is that the bodies of these rats were not satisfied due to the vitamin deficiency: they had an established reflex which equated enough food (calories) with enough other nutrients, and they were hungry since they were not able to metabolize their food as well. Whenever I have an hyperactive child in my office and I see his or her agitated behavior, I am reminded of this experiment and I think that the child's body, due to the deficiency of certain B vitamins, is compelled to respond as did the rats kept on a B vitamin deficient diet. I think it is a reasonable hypothesis that patients with eating disorders also are trying to obtain enough nutrients by increasing the amount of food they eat, but the major increase in calories which drives them to obesity forces them to seek ways of controlling the food intake by vomiting or using laxatives. With vomiting they do not get any extra nutrients, but with the laxatives they may obtain a few more of the essential nutrients they would otherwise not obtain. It is probable that all the addictions are caused by similar factors — by the excessive intake of

LAW

I think it is a reasonable hypothesis that patients with eating disorders also are trying to obtain enough nutrients by increasing the amount of food they eat, but the major increase in calories which drives them to obesity forces them to seek ways of controlling the food intake by vomiting or using laxatives.

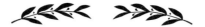

sugars and starches combined with the deficiency of essential nutrients.

The main diseases of the esophagus and stomach are hiatus hernia, dyspepsia, peptic ulcer, and cancer. With respect to hiatus hernia there are two main symptoms, the discomfort after meals which is often confused with dyspepsia, and the actual bulging of the esophageal-gastric juncture through the diaphragm. The pain and discomfort comes from the high sugar, low fat diet, especially if the patient is allergic to these foods. Many of my patients, who had been diagnosed as having hiatus hernia by their physicians, lost all their discomfort when the foods they were allergic to were eliminated from the diet. The bulging is caused by the constipation and the frequent straining the patient has to do to have bowel movements.

Ulcer is caused by eating foods which are too low in fiber and in protein. When we start to eat, the stomach prepares to do its job of secreting hydrochloric acid needed before pepsin can digest protein. When the food enters the stomach, the acid is absorbed onto the protein and cannot do any harm to the walls of the stomach. The acidity in the stomach can be very high, so high that if you put your finger into stomach contents it will be burned. The stomach wall can resist the acid which it secretes but not if it lays about in the stomach too long. If one drinks a soft drink which contains no protein and which is already high in acid, there will be nothing there to absorb the acid and it will damage the stomach wall. Not all high protein foods are useful. If the high protein food in itself stimulates the extra secretion of acid, it will have a detrimental effect. This is one of the problems with dairy products. It is odd but many years ago the favorite treatment for peptic ulcer was the high milk diet called the Sippi diet. It is now known that people with peptic ulcers ought to avoid milk. Antacids decrease the secretion of acid and are useful in the treatment of peptic ulcers. Niacin may also increase the secretion of acid but it can also

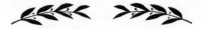

absorb some acid. A few patients with ulcer cannot tolerate it but most of the patients I have treated, who had ulcers, were able to take niacin with no difficulty. It did not increase their pain and discomfort. Fiber can also absorb acid and in this way prevent it from attacking the stomach wall. The most recent clinical evidence is strong that most cases of peptic ulcer are caused by a bacterium, helicobacter pylorii. Specific treatment with a proper antibiotic regimen will cure most of them. Chronic infection in combination with a poor diet is the main factor. Peptic ulcer will appear with either factor alone, but is more more likely when both are present, and is best treated by using both the diet as described here and the correct antibiotic treatment. There is recent evidence that the chronic infection — that is, chronic peptic ulcer — is a predisposing factor for stomach cancer.

The cause of cancer of the stomach is not as clear. Malnutrition is a major factor because of the deficiency of antioxidants such as vitamin C, vitamin E, selenium, and others. It is known that chronic irritation of any tissue is also one of the factors. For this reason, a chronic peptic ulcer in a person also suffering shortages of essential micro nutrients is more susceptible to the development of cancer.

The major part of the digestion, the breaking down of the food into its primary components, occurs in the small intestine and partially in the large intestine or colon. For this there was must be an adequate supply of enzymes from the pancreas and from the intestinal walls; and there must be enough muscular movement to propel the intestinal contents slowly towards the rectum. The movement is called peristalsis and consists of alternate contraction and dilation, like squeezing a tooth paste container to expel the contents. When the foods remain undigested and when there is too little bulk or fiber, the intestine and colon have great difficulty in performing their main function. This results in a number of pathological changes which have been considered separate diseases but are really various expressions of

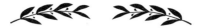

the one disease, the Saccharine Disease.

The main symptom arising from lack of fiber is constipation because the intestinal walls are not challenged by the lack of bulk in the food. The muscular walls apparently have to have some stimulus which comes from the extension of the diameter of the bowel by the accumulation of food therein. As a result of the constipation which is usually chronic and may be very severe other symptoms develop. Because of the need to strain to eliminate the stools, there is more back pressure on the veins around the anus and this will result in hemorrhoids if the problem is there for a long time. With chronic constipation there may be a large amount of fecal material in the colon which exerts pressure on the large veins leading from the legs to the heart. When this is present long enough it may lead to varicous veins in people who are, for reasons not known, more susceptible to this vascular problem. The increased back pressure may also lead to small bulgings in the wall of the intestine called diverticulosis, and if these become infected, they are called diverticulitis. Appendicitis is also considered one of the consequences. It was known in South Africa many years ago that only people who spoke English ever got appendicitis. This was because they were eating the low fiber diet which was responsible for this. The increased back pressure may also lead to gall bladder disease, according to the same authors. Finally there is an increased likelihood of getting cancer of the colon due to the combination of poor nutrition and back pressure.

When too much sugar is present it will be absorbed into the blood stream too quickly and compromise the ability of the body to deal with these amounts. The body is used to absorbing the sugar slowly as it is released from its foods by digestion. If the sugar cannot all be absorbed, it will find its way down to the colon where there should not be any and provide food for organisms that should not be there such as the yeasts. Undigested sugars too far into the colon will create serious problems. A good example is the lactose in

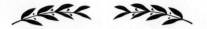

milk, milk sugar. This is a double sugar, a disaccharide, consisting of a union between one glucose molecule and one galactose molecule. In infants and to a lesser degree in children and adults, the stomach provides the enzyme lactase which splits this sugar in the intestine. But when it is lacking, as it is in many adults, the original sugar passes down until it can be fermented by the fungi and yeast in the colon and create serious symptoms of diarrhea, gas, pain, and so on. This problem is solved by swallowing lactase tablets (the enzyme) at the same time one drinks the milk. If sucrose (common table sugar which is also a double sugar made from glucose and fructose) is not split, a similar problem will develop.

Overloading with sugar throws an extra burden on the pancreas to release enough insulin to deal with the amount absorbed. This is stressful to the pancreas. There is a direct association between the annual consumption of all the sugars and the incidence of diabetes mellitus. T.L. Cleave in his book *The Saccharine Disease* pointed this out some time ago. He formulated the 20 year rule — it takes about 20 years after any group of people go onto the high sugar diet before it begins to show up in the statistics. In Canada the incidence of diabetes has risen from around one percent fifty years ago when I took my medical training to about four percent today. In some countries, for example in Mexico, the incidence is very much higher and some epidemiologists have complained that about 40 per cent of the population are potentially diabetic.

Of course the intake of sugars is not the only factor in causing diabetes. Evidence is accumulating that viral infections can destroy the Islets of Langerhans in the pancreas and this can be a main problem, even for people who do not eat much sugar. Genes have been found in some families which are possibly causal, but there is striking evidence that taking niacinamide will protect them from getting diabetes. In fact niacin and niacinamide (vitamin B-3) has

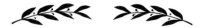

valuable healing properties for every organ in the body, including the pancreas and kidneys.

Excessive intake of sugars is much more closely related to relative hypoglycemia. This is measured by the standard five hour glucose tolerance test. The normal curve present for healthy people is distorted for people with high sugar diets, usually by going too high in the first two or three hours and then dipping down too quickly and too far over the last two or three hours. People with this problem often note an exacerbation of symptoms such as drowsiness, sleepiness, nausea, and headache a few hours after meals rich in the sugars. It is found in almost every person who is obese. Many doctors do not read the last two hours, however, and if the first three hours are normal will conclude that the entire test curve is normal. They will advise patients that they do not have this condition of hypoglycemia and may also advise them to control their low blood sugar by taking more sugar. This is inappropriate advice since it is the sugar intake that was responsible for the drop in sugar. Other foods will also yield similar low blood sugars if the person is allergic to these foods. Hypoglycemia is found most frequently in middle-aged obese patients and may be confused with diabetes. They usually respond well to dietary control and do not require insulin.

Vascular disease caused by arteriosclerosis is a very common and serious outcome of the low fiber, high sugar diet. I will not discuss this in any detail since it is an enormous problem. The current idea is that the fat intake of the diet is the main factor in causing elevated cholesterol levels with the resultant increase in hardening of the arteries. The debate is growing and vigorous with many more now maintaining that fat in the diet is not the main factor. Investigators are examining the connection between vessel disease and the

> *I am convinced that high sugar intake is a greater risk factor for heart disease than is the fat level of the food.*

LAW

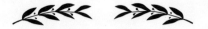

total fat, the type of fat, the ratio of cholesterol to high density lipo protein cholesterol, and so on. Unfortunately very few are looking at the sugar intake, especially sucrose. It is clear that people on a low fat diet will increase their sugar intake unless they are advised not to do so. If they do, any gain they might obtain by lowering fat will be overcome by the increased pathological effect of sugar on cholesterol levels. This area of research will have to be studied much more carefully. I am convinced that high sugar intake is a greater risk factor for heart disease than is the fat level of the food. The low fat diets which are rich in complex carbohydrates and are low in sugar should be the best diet for preventing arteriosclerosis.

Ulcerative colitis and Crohns disease are also symptoms of the high sugar, low fiber diet, according to T.L. Cleave. I have treated many patients with Crohns disease and find that many of them are allergic to wheat and other grains and to dairy products. Dairy foods, considered by many physicians and nutritionists to be an essential food group, are in fact the cause of allergies and disease in many people.

FOOD ALLERGIES

Dairy Products

The most informative single study that describes dairy products and human nutrition is Frank Oski's book entitled *Don't Drink Your Milk*. Milk and its many derivatives are the most widely promoted and advertised food product in North America and major parts of Europe. According to Dr. Oski, at the time his book was written, 14 percent of all food dollars went for milk and its products. This made up the second major food expense following the combined costs of meat, fish, poultry, and eggs. These products are promoted by the vast majority of physicians, by almost every dietitian and nutritionist, by most professors of nutrition and biochemistry when they teach nutrition in medical schools, by

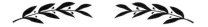

Departments of Public Health, and of course by the most powerful group of all, the various national, provincial, and state dairy organizations. It has become an article of faith that unless children are given copious quantities of milk, best of all three glasses each day, they will not grow, they will not develop, their babies will not get enough calcium, and the women will all get osteoporosis after their menopause.

> *I believe we should have different names for human milk and for cow milk so that they will not be equated as equivalent good products. Cow milk is good for calves but has never been shown by any independent experiment to be good for human babies or for adult women to protect them against osteoporosis.*

LAW

I invariably get a startled reaction from mothers when I advise them their children or even they must stop drinking milk. The first question is where will I get enough calcium, how about osteoporosis. The public is confused about the various mammalian milks. I believe we should have different names for human milk and for cow milk so that they will not be equated as equivalent good products. Cow milk is good for calves but has never been shown by any independent experiment to be good for human babies or for adult women to protect them against osteoporosis. Against the position taken by the dairy industry are a few dedicated individual physicians such as Dr. Oski and a growing band of supporters who maintain that milk is not a perfect food, that it is not even a good food, and that milk must be used with extreme caution. I would support the idea that all dairy products be labeled with the warning sign applied to cigarette packages, something like *Warning, This Product May Be Hazardous to Your Health.*

Most mammal's feed on their mothers milk until they have tripled their birth weight. In human infants, this takes about one year. From all the mammals the human species alone never gets weaned from milk. Since formula is rich in sugar and milk is rich in lactose (another sugar), it is more

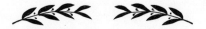

accurate to say that only humans never get weaned from milk and sugar. As will become clear later these are two of the most common and most injurious food allergens. Americans and many Europeans have developed a taste for milk which is not natural, while most people in East Asia, Africa, and South America regard milk as not fit for human consumption. They are in better tune with the rest of our mammalian cousins. We have broken the adaptation between our need and the food by depending so much on cow milk. Nature never intended that children should forever be dependent on their mother's milk, and the loss of the enzyme lactase is a reflection of this adaptation.

<blockquote>
LAW

I would support the idea that all dairy products be labeled with the warning sign applied to cigarette packages, something like Warning, This Product May Be Hazardous to Your Health.
</blockquote>

Milk causes the following reactions in human subjects: gastrointestinal disturbances arising from lactose intolerance and from milk allergies, and nutrient deficiencies arising from these gastrointestinal reactions. It plays a role in the development of atherosclerosis and may play a role in the development of childhood leukemia, multiple sclerosis, and tooth decay in infants. It plays an epidemiological role in cancer, and is involved as one of the causal factors in children and adults in antisocial and criminal behavior.

Gastrointestinal disorders may be due to lactose intolerance. After infancy, many people no longer make enough lactase, the enzyme that splits lactose into galactose and glucose. The lactose cannot be absorbed and stays in the intestine where it is fermented by bacteria creating a lot of gas and intense bowel discomfort. The frequency of lactase deficiency varies enormously between various peoples. Over 80 percent of Filipinos, Japanese, Taiwanese, and Thais lack this enzyme. Over 60 percent of Blacks, Arabs, Jews, and Greek Cypriots also lack this enzyme, while under 10 percent of

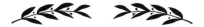

Danes, Swiss, and American Whites have the same problem. Peoples that had to depend upon milk to survive have by a process of natural selection retained the ability to create lactase long after it was natural for the same people who did not have to consume so much. Thus in Nigeria, tribes that did not raise cattle had a 99 percent deficiency of lactase, while other tribes where milk was a traditional food had only a 20 percent lactase deficiency. This is good news for the dairy industry, for if milk consumption can be maintained long enough, no matter what the cost, most groups will have developed the ability to retain lactase production. However, it is now possible to swallow lactase tablets before the milk is drunk and to drink lactase treated milk and thus avoid most of the symptoms of lactase deficiency.

This will not solve the problem for the milk allergic individual. For allergic reactions to dairy products are very common and can cause an amazing variety of allergic reactions anywhere in the gastrointestinal tract and very often in the upper respiratory system. I am an expert in dairy allergy, one among many, because I have a fixed allergy to these foods. Many years ago I got a common cold, at least that is what I thought it was. I did what I should have done to bring it under control, including taking large quantities of vitamin C and vitamin A, but there was no relief. For two years I had a constant nasal drip which was so bad that when I gave a lecture I would have to hold a kleenex in one hand and my notes in the other. I always carried pockets full of kleenex. After two years I had given up hope. At that time, for other reasons, I did a four-day water fast. To my amazement, I was well by the fourth day. On a retest with a little milk my drippy nose promptly returned in about 15 minutes. For the next few years, whenever I was exposed to dairy products, whether I was aware of it or not, I would get another four-day cold. Since then, for about 35 years, I have not had any colds and have been inadvertently exposed to dairy foods only on a few occasions. My dairy allergy

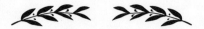

expressed itself as a runny nose, congested sinuses, sore throat, with difficulty in clearing my ears with changes in air pressure.

The most common gastrointestinal reaction is chronic diarrhea, ranging from frequent soft stools to numerous, watery, explosive stools, occasionally showing traces of red blood. The diarrhea impairs the absorption of nutrients. If there is chronic slow bleeding, a protein deficiency will develop leading to swelling of the abdomen, hands, and feet. It will also lead to iron deficiency. Half the iron deficiency in infants is a result of feeding infants cow milk. Iron deficiency will make many babies irritable with impaired attention span. This has caused a common problem called the "blue bottle syndrome." The child walks about with a plastic bottle of milk from which he drinks now and then. When only glass bottles were available they would drop these so often and break them that mothers would stop giving them bottles. With plastic bottles there is no relief for the child. Blue bottle babies are usually iron deficient. Colic is a common manifestation of milk allergy. In adults peptic ulcer is another reaction. There are too many different reactions to list them here. Any good book on clinical ecology will describe these in detail.

Dairy allergy is present in a considerably high percentage of the North American population. Dr. J. Gerrard, Professor of Pediatrics at the Medical School, University of Saskatchewan, after a series of careful studies, concluded that 59 infants out of 787 were milk allergic, or 7.5 percent. He reported that the frequency depended upon how soon the infants were started on milk. One quarter of the babies started on milk before they were three months became milk allergic. Milk allergy causes nephrosis, eczema, growing pains, rheumatoid arthritis, appendicitis, and predisposes one to Group A beta-hemolytic streptococcus infection.

The psychiatric and behavioral changes caused by milk

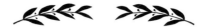

are also numerous. Any food allergy can cause almost every known psychiatric syndrome and milk is no exception. The first dramatic case I saw was a teenaged girl who was typically schizophrenic with visual and auditory hallucinations, many paranoid delusions, and severe depression. She had not responded to any previous treatment. But after a four-day water fast she was normal. One day later after one glass of milk she was psychotic again in one hour. I have also seen a chronic paranoid schizophrenic who had been resident in a mental hospital for years. He suddenly could not urinate. He was brought to City Hospital in Saskatoon from the mental hospital and came under my care when it was found he was physically normal. After a fast he was normal. The next day after a test dose of milk, he became violently ill with nausea, vomiting, severe diarrhea, headache, and more. He had been mentally normal after the fast but after milk he was once more the same psychotic person I had known for many years. The case ended sadly. He refused to keep away from dairy products because, he told me, if he remained well he would have to get a job and try to make his way outside the hospital. He was too old for this and preferred to remain in a mental hospital where he would be looked after. He died there two years later from leukemia.

Over a period of about three years I fasted over 100 patients who had not responded or had responded only partially to the treatment I was using. More than 75 percent were much better after the four-day fast. Of these many were milk allergic. The syndromes produced by these allergies included learning and behavioral disorders, depressions, and schizophrenias. One female had been depressed for over 20 years. She had not been helped by medication or even one series of electro-convulsive treatment. She went onto a dairy free diet on a Friday and by the following Monday her depression was gone. When I take a history I never forget to take an allergy history in the hunt for clues. With children

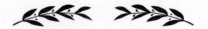

or young adults it is vital to examine for the presence of the common allergic diseases as a factor in causing their psychiatric problems.

As well as causing iron deficiency due to chronic bleeding in the gut, excessive intake of milk also is associated with other nutrient deficiencies. Excessive intake of dairy products crowds other foods out of the diet, foods which are richer in vitamins and minerals. Another factor is chronic inflammation of the intestine which decreases absorption of nutrients. I have already referred to protein deficiency caused by the milk. Another common deficiency is zinc and pyridoxine. I have been surprised at the large number of children I have seen who had white areas in their finger nails. This is due to a deficiency of pyridoxine and zinc. Most often these children are heavy consumers of dairy products. In some cases 50 percent of their calories came from this source. Milk tends to be low in zinc and in pyridoxine.

There are many nutrient deficiencies involved in the production of atherosclerosis, including deficiencies in ascorbic acid, nicotinic acid, and pyridoxine. Excess intake of sugar as well as excess consumption of fat calories are important factors as well. The major source of excess calories in the human diet comes from dairy products. Early consumption of milk is associated with atherosclerosis. A pathologist examined the coronary arteries from 1500 children and adolescents who had died as a result of accident. Some of the children had normal blood vessels, others did not. The single characteristic that distinguished them was that the children whose arteries were not normal had been fed cow milk or formula based on dairy products.

The Lancet, a British medical journal, reported some years ago that unpasteurized milk fed to six baby chimpanzees caused two of them to develop leukemia. The milk had come from infected cows with bovine C-type virus. Later *Science* carried a report written by three doctors from University of Pennsylvania, School of Veterinary Medicine.

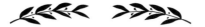

They concluded that there was an association between human and bovine leukemia, that there was a significant increase in the number of humans with acute lymphoid leukemia in areas with a high incidence of bovine leukemia. They suggested that there must be further investigation of this relationship. Very few people drink unpasteurized milk in high-tech societies. This will be a problem for countries that do not pasteurize their milk.

Two scientists from the University of Michigan began to look for links between multiple sclerosis and environmental factors. They found a striking correlation between the incidence of multiple sclerosis and low per capita milk consumption in the United States. The correlation was 0.82. In Europe a similar relationship was found. Patients with M.S. do very much better when they are on a low fat diet. A low fat diet means that dairy products are eliminated from it, as they are the major source of fats. Dr. R.L. Swank and his colleagues have found that patients with M.S. who adhered to his low fat diet regimen, described in his *The Multiple Sclerosis Diet Book,* had the best results. Patients who started on the program early had the best results. Swank also saw a cultural and demographic pattern linked to the incidence of M.S. As he explains, "two parallel and little mixed cultures based on food have evolved. These are the beer-butter and the wine-oil cultures. The first extended across northern Europe (Scandinavia, Germany, Holland, Belgium, northern France, northern Switzerland, and the British Isles) and has become the mode of life in the United States and Canada. The second predominates in the Mediterranean area (Spain, Italy, southern France, southern Switzerland, and Greece) and stretches to the Middle East and North Africa. The beer-butter culture corresponds geographically to the area of high incidence of multiple sclerosis and vascular disease; the wine-oil culture corresponds to the area where these conditions have a low incidence." Of course there are other factors as well. M.S. is caused by environmental factors in

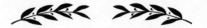

genetically susceptible individuals. It is important that these various factors be isolated and their relative importance in the cause and in the treatment be examined. In the meantime the optimum diet for patients with multiple sclerosis is the Swank diet.

Many neurologists are not aware of Dr. Swank's findings, or if they are, they ignore them as being too simple. They are, however, keenly interested in drug treatment, and when they have a drug that has any therapeutic properties whatever, no matter how little, they become very enthusiastic. In the Toronto *Globe and Mail* it was recently reported that beta interferon was being recommended for sale in the U.S.A. as a treatment for M.S. A Canadian neurologist researching M.S. for many years was reported to have said, "I'm a little cynical about anything that claims to do something. I've done a lot of these trials. But when I saw these results they blew my mind. Talk to anyone in the M.S. field today and they're just ecstatic. It's not that the drug makes people get better. People will still get worse, but not at the same rate." The cost was $5,000 to $7,000 per year for this injectable drug. The drug was tested only on the patients who had not become irreversibly ill. I find it very difficult to understand the enthusiasm for an expensive drug which is less effective than placing these good prognostic patients on a simple low fat diet as recommended by Dr. Swank. A combination of this diet plus vitamins has been very successful in my patients, and I have seen many who have gotten well, or if they have not, they have stopped deteriorating and are neurologically stable. Vitamin C is a natural booster of interferon production in the body and has been shown to double the concentration.

Dr. F. Castano, a research dentist, has evidence that milk will increase tooth decay. Many mothers use milk to get their babies to fall asleep. The baby sucks at the bottle and dozes off. The baby stops swallowing the milk, which then stays in the mouth and begins to eat away at the teeth. During sleep saliva production is decreased. The milk on the teeth turns

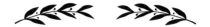

sour, by the same bacteria which causes dental caries. Dr. Castano has observed that decay has been so rapid that the teeth appeared to be melting away, especially if the milk drinking practice is continued after age 12 months. Juices in bottles are just as bad. Babies should not be put to bed with a bottle in their mouth.

Of all the possible connections between cancer and diet the one most readily accepted by the cancer research agencies is the relationship to fat. There is almost a linear relationship between the average fat consumption of the diet of various countries and the incidence of breast cancer. In the United States and Canada and many European countries 40 percent of calories come from fat. These countries have the highest incidence of breast cancer. Countries where fat intake is below 10 percent have a much lower incidence. There is also a direct link between fat consumption and estrogen secretion. Women eating high fat diets secrete more estrogen.

Any food allergy can reproduce almost every known psychiatric syndrome from infantile autism and schizophrenia to mood and behavioral disorders. I do not single milk out as the only villain in the production of allergic reactions. Allergic reactions tend to develop against staple foods. Thus in wheat consuming countries, wheat allergy is much more common than it is in rice consuming countries where rice is a greater problem. In tea drinking countries, tea will more often cause allergic reactions than coffee, while the converse is true in coffee consuming countries. I have seldom seen allergic reactions to tea but coffee allergic reactions are more common in Canada. Milk is a major staple since almost every one is introduced to it early, either directly or via their mothers who drink milk, and it is consumed for a long time.

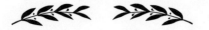

For this reason milk allergy is a major problem and amongst the allergic reactions it induces, the psychiatric ones are common. They include behavioral and learning disorders in children. I had one young boy as a patient who in the fall was at the bottom of his class of 20. On a milk free diet he was at the top by the following spring. Another youngster diagnosed with infantile autism by a clinic specializing in these disorders became normal on a diet free of dairy and sugar products in one month. His mother had placed him on this diet against the advice of his therapists, who laughed at her when she first discussed it with them.

The vast majority of people in North America and in Europe can consume dairy products with few problems, especially those who have been consuming it for many centuries, because they have been adapted to this as a major food supply. Others can use it in small amounts with no harm, but for those who suffer any of the above conditions milk is as poisonous as any other food causing similar reactions would be. The active defence of dairy products by the dairy industry dismisses airily the findings of legitimate research scientists and nutritionists, including the eminent pediatrician Dr. B. Spock. The Dairy Bureau of Canada labels him a "radical animal-rights activist," thus dismissing his attempts to improve our health. This arrogant dismissal of the harm caused by dairy products to many people will simply delay recognition by many patients that they are sick because they cannot tolerate dairy products.

Processed Protein

For many decades protein has been looked upon as something we should all have in ample quantities. Like motherhood, little bad could be said against protein. But the term should be applied only to protein-rich foods, not to the pure protein which is extracted from food and then used to make artificial products or artifacts. The natural diet will provide ample protein in its original form. Seldom

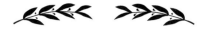

do people need more than that. High protein diets can be tolerated provided this means high protein-rich foods, but there is no advantage to this diet and there may be a number of disadvantages. A high protein diet increases the demand for calcium and is one of the factors leading to osteoporosis. Foods prepared from processed meat and fish are not as nutritious as the original food and ought not to be used as food. This includes extruded proteins, whether of animal or vegetable origin. It includes imitation fish, such as processed lobster or other artifacts which look like and try to taste like the original fish but seldom succeed.

> *High protein diets can be tolerated provided this means high protein-rich foods, but there is no advantage to this diet and there may be a number of disadvantages.*

LAW

Several years ago there was some interest in converting oil to protein and then using this as food. Maybe one day when we know much much more about nutrition and our needs it may be possible to make synthetic food identical to the food to which we had adapted. But that time has not yet come. At the beginning of the twentieth century nutritionists in England were convinced that only protein, fat, and carbohydrate were important for human nutrition. Baby foods were then prepared from this formula, but babies who were fed this artificial product to meet their nutritional needs died. It appears to me we have not yet learned anything from this gross experiment with human infants or from other attempts to replace alive, whole, and fresh food with artifacts.

PUBLIC
MALNUTRITION

❦

A recent report in the Proceedings of the National Academy of Science, reviewed in the Toronto *Globe and Mail* in 1993, described how the people living in the "Biosphere 2" environmental project depended on food grown in the Biosphere. They planned on living there for two years sealed so that only sunlight, electrical energy, and heat was allowed to exchange with the outside environment. This was a model of a closed ecosystem. The diet consisted of fresh fruits, cereals, peas, peanuts, beans, greens, sweet and white potatoes, with small quantities of goat milk and yogurt, goat meat, pork, chicken, fish, and eggs. Vitamins and minerals were taken as well. The fat intake was 10 percent of the total calories. They entered the biosphere 26 September 1991. At the time of the report they were well. After six months they discovered that they needed only 1780 calories per day instead of the usual 2500 North Americans consume. They exercised a lot and worked three to four hours each day. Their weight decreased by 12 kilograms for the men and 7 for the women. Their mean blood pressure dropped 20 percent, mean blood sugar by 18 percent, and mean blood cholesterol by 36 percent.

Dr. Colin Rose, cardiologist and associate professor of medicine at McGill University who was the senior author of

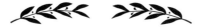

the report in the *Globe and Mail,* said, "This is astounding. Conventional Western medical wisdom dictates that only 5 to 10 percent of blood cholesterol can be influenced by diet, and that only rare 'salt sensitive' people will change their blood pressures minimally on a low-salt diet. Most physicians we know believe that these parameters are genetically determined and can be altered only with drugs, if at all."

Dr. R. Walford, one of the "citizens" in the Biosphere, makes the point that if all Americans were to follow this diet the U.S.A. would save $50 billion dollars per year from the remarkable caloric reduction, about $100 billion per year from the decreased need of packaging for processed foods no longer used, and $200 billion per year from savings gained through the decreased incidence of diseases caused by the typical high-tech diet and through the decrease in the amount of drugs needed. Oral hypoglycemics, cholesterol lowering drugs, blood pressure lowering drugs, and treatment for obesity account for billions of dollars. Preventing these would prevent their complications, such as blindness, renal failure, heart attacks, heart failure, blocked leg arteries, and strokes. In short the Biosphere scientists have found exactly what orthomolecular nutritionists have been claiming. They confirmed data gathered by all the nutritionists who actually did field work and studied the diet and health of primitive people everywhere, before they came into contact with the nutritional habits of high-tech society. Of course a change of the national diet towards what the citizens of the Biosphere consumed would produce a major translocation of the entire food and agricultural complex and will be resisted by industry and the labor unions alike for this reason. I believe a lot of the gross national product depends upon the creation of disease by

I believe a lot of the gross national product depends upon the creation of disease by the high-tech diet and the treatment of its symptoms by the huge medical and pharmaceutical establishment.

LAW

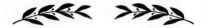

the high-tech diet and the treatment of its symptoms by the huge medical and pharmaceutical establishment.

HEALTH CARE CRISIS

Canada's universal health care programs were introduced many years ago, before there was enough information on which to base the future cost of disease. No consideration was given to the impact of the high-tech diet on the production of ill health. If the prevalence and incidence of disease had remained constant at the 1960 level, there would be no economic crises in health care. Professor Brian Ferguson, Associate Professor of Economics at the University of Guelph, Ontario, has been studying the cost-effectiveness of health care in Canada. In the *Globe and Mail* on 22 March 1993 he reported that the Canadian system in comparison to the one in the U.S.A. has not "enabled us to control the growth of health-care costs." The cost of physician services had risen faster in Canada than it had in the U.S.A. He pointed out that the health care system of both countries yielded similar results if measured by the usual measures, such as infant mortality. I do not think any health care system which ignores the profound effect of nutrition of health and disease is going to make any appreciable difference to the general health of any nation. Modern medicine has gone as far as it can with its present methodology and therapeutic measures and there it will stay until nutrition is brought into the body of medicine, taught in medical schools, and used by the profession.

In my opinion, there has been a real increase in the number of people who become sick, despite the ever increasing amount of money spent to make them well. Secondary costs are generated by improved methods of diagnosing and treating. But these costs are not the main reason, nor is inflation the main culprit, since the proportion of the gross national product consumed by costs of treating disease remains about the same. Today every second Canadian has

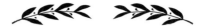

one or more degenerative disease. Nor is it to be blamed on the increase in the average age of our population. It is not necessary for people who age to become sick. Large numbers of old people remain well and do not burden the health care system. The reasons so many do, however, are the same as those which cause even children to become ill. This massive increase in disease related costs has occurred coincidentally with many remarkable improvements in treating and preventing disease. We no longer have major epidemics of pellagra or scurvy, or of some of the infectious diseases so common in the past. Any rational person would have predicted on the basis of what has been discovered that our society would be much healthier and our citizens would live much longer — and that costs would have gone down substantially. Why, then, has just the reverse occurred? On the average people live longer, that is, many more live into old age, but the expectation of additional years by the time one reaches 50 has not changed in the past 100 years. What has gone wrong? Why did we not foresee these changes in 1960 when our health plans were being formulated?

> *Modern medicine has gone as far as it can with its present methodology and therapeutic measures and there it will stay until nutrition is brought into the body of medicine, taught in medical schools, and used by the profession.*

LAW

In my opinion, the planners did not foresee the impact on health of the major technological changes in our food supply. I am convinced the rapid deterioration of the quality of our food is the major factor in causing our health crisis today. Twenty-five years ago the evidence connecting the quality of our food and health was not as well known. There were many individual physicians and people interested in nutrition who did understand and warned us but no one listened. Today the evidence is available to a much larger degree: it is clear and striking, yet it is still consistently ignored by the medical profession and governments responsible for administering public health and food quality measures. Canadian medical

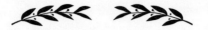

schools neglect to teach their students the importance of good nutrition in treating disease and maintaining health. When they do attempt to teach nutrition, it is left to biochemists who are not clinicians — they have never seen the impact of poor food in causing disease and of good food in restoring health. The American medical schools are no better.

> **LAW** *I am convinced the rapid deterioration of the quality of our food is the major factor in causing our health crisis today.*

The first major studies of the link between health and nutrition arose out of the two world wars. Due to trade blockades, England was not able to provide the same diet to the people. The per capita consumption of sugar decreased from about 120 pounds per person per year to half that amount. There was also a major decrease in the use of white flour and meat. White flour was replaced by a longer extraction (browner), more nutritious flour containing more wheat germ and bran, and vegetables were used more. The government carried out a massive educational campaign to teach the people how to make nourishing meals from their vegetables. Governments in Canada and the United States consider we are in a health crisis today. Perhaps they should study the English model and follow the methods the English were forced to use by their war crisis. We have an equally important war to wage against disease.

Physicians, especially psychiatrists, had predicted with great confidence that there would be a major increase in disease in England due to the stress of war, the bombing, the dislocations of people, the loss of homes, the deprivations. It was predicted there would be a major increase in the psychosomatic diseases such as peptic ulcer, ulcerative colitis, arthritis, thyroid disease, and more. But after the war, to everyone's surprise, it was found that none of the predictions had come true. On the contrary, the people as a whole had never been healthier. There was a major decrease in disease, even in psychiatric disease. For the first time there was

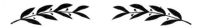

a decrease in the incidence of schizophrenia as well as in heart disease and peptic ulcer. After the war the government discontinued the educational program, removed the wartime restriction on the importation of sugar and white flour, and the intake of sugar quickly returned to the previous 120 pounds per year.

Other countries with similar drastic changes in their food consumption experienced similar vast improvement in their overall health. Denmark enforced a major reduction in animal food plus other changes. They decreased sugar, became more vegetarian, and became much healthier.

Epidemiological studies of people who have forsaken their native diet have invariably found an increase in ill health. In South Africa, the prevalence of diabetes and cancer of the colon was very low as long as the inhabitants lived on their native high fiber, low sugar diets. As these people adopted the modern high sugar, low fiber diet they have become very ill. In Israel about 40 years ago, Jews from North Africa were examined and found to be physically healthy, free of modern disease. Today the same people are suffering from as much disease as their fellow citizens. It takes about 20 years of the high-tech diet for the high-tech diseases to develop.

Animal studies have shown that once a population of animals is placed upon an inadequate diet, the health of the animals decreased for eight generations when it reached a steady state of poor health. If the diet is restored to the level which had maintained good health in the past, it required another four generations before the original state of health was achieved. To compare this with what happens to human populations, let us accept that one generation is about 20 years. If the animals studies are significant, we will continue to deteriorate for 160 years if our diet is maintained at its present poor level. The animal studies did not reproduce what has happened to us because our diet has not remained at a steady poor state. It has been deteriorating

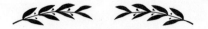

over the past 100 years. It would therefore appear probable that the deterioration of our general health will accelerate. In any event, we might expect to achieve a steady state of miserable health in about 160 years. Perhaps we will reach a state where 90 percent of the population has one or more chronic disease. Dating the beginning of the massive change in our food supply around 1940, we can expect to continue to deteriorate until about 2100 A.D. If, however, we learn the lesson of what has happened and get back onto the diet to which we have adapted it will take another 80 years(four generations) before we regain the state of health we had before we embarked on the massive deterioration experiment. However, I think the process of recovery can be greatly accelerated by taking ample quantities of the nutrients on which our high-tech diets have made us dependent.

IRRESPONSIBLE MEDICINE

D.C. Hemingway has recently examined the relationship of good nutrition to health costs. He refers to other recent studies where the amount of disease caused by poor nutrition has been studied primarily in institutions such as hospitals and nursing homes. These are the last places in the world one would expect nutrition to be so totally neglected. In one study it was found that many patients in a local hospital suffered from protein-calorie malnutrition. Half the surgical patients suffered and the medical patients were even worse off. In another study, 20 percent of the patients studied were deficient in each nutrient examined, even though some of the normal controls had very low values for the same nutrients. I am not surprised. I attended one of the hospital staff meetings where the budget was analyzed. To my amazement, that hospital spent more on bandages and plaster casts than it had for food for the year. Diabetics, who generally are more nutrition conscious, had fewer deficiencies, while peptic ulcer patients had the lowest vitamin C

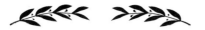

levels. In general malnutrition was widespread. Here are some other surprising statistics:

- 31% of 200 consecutive patients were malnourished on admission.
- 65% of 1000 surgical patients in an affluent suburban hospital had moderate to severe malnutrition.
- 100 % of the malnourished patients who received no nutritional support for three weeks in hospital experienced deterioration of their nutritional status. They were more malnourished after spending three weeks in a modern hospital.
- 75% of well nourished patients who were hospitalized for two weeks or longer showed a decline in their nutritional status.
- Malnourished patients stayed 90% longer in hospital than other medical patients.
- Malnourished patients had 75% higher costs of care compared with the overall hospital average.

The amount of malnutrition is just as bad in nursing homes. In one home with 232 patients, 59 percent of the patients showed some protein-calorie malnutrition. Seventeen had bed sores — they were all in the severely malnourished group. Another study showed that 60,000 deaths each year in the United States came from skin destructive bed sores.

Dr. Hemingway has proposed "that we as Canadians and Governments must improve the nutritional status of Canadians to lower our health care costs. Governments can demonstrate the effectiveness of nutrition by promoting better nutrition for our hospital patients. Governments could recognize nutrition therapy fees under 'medicare' and as income tax deductions. This would encourage doctors and patients to use nutrition instead of drugs. Governments on behalf of the people of Canada must take the initiative to

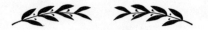

finance studies to show the effectiveness of Nutritional Therapy and Nutrition as a method of disease prevention. Industry cannot finance nutrition research because their shareholders demand profits. Nutrients cannot be patented and therefore there is no way to recover the costs of the research. Insurance companies, governments and citizens are the people that pay medical bills and they are the ones that can benefit from lower health care costs. We as health professionals and concerned citizens must continue to encourage our politicians to take a more active role in Health Maintenance."

Dr. Hemingway concluded his excellent report by quoting from Dr. T.D. Spies, in an article published in the *Journal of the American Medical Association* in 1958. Dr Spies was one of the foremost nutritional physicians of the times, an expert pellagrologist and clinical nutritionist: "I have discussed with you a few of the many advances which have been made in nutrition in recent years. You have seen that what patients eat has much to do with their health and with their recovery from ill health. Primary or secondary nutritional disorders produce or complicate all the problems of the sick. I have stressed that we should be concerned with the prevention and with the earlier stages of disease when the disturbances are almost imperceptible and that we should not wait until these disturbances bring tremendous burdens and stark tragedies."

The above quotation is as applicable today as when it was written over 30 years ago. It is sad that we learn so slowly, that pride keeps us from accepting the discoveries and teachings of our colleagues. We cannot change the past but we can use the information gleaned from the past to change our ways of promoting health today. Tomorrow is our responsibility.

Modern food technology has become food chemistry. We know a good deal about the chemical structure of food.

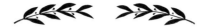

But in the process of developing the chemistry of food we have neglected to study the physiology of food; there is thus an almost total imbalance between our needs and what we eat. It is almost as odd as feeding lions only on grass. Our needs are the type of whole foods to which our ancestors had adapted 10,000 years ago. Since then we have remained the same physiologically but our food supply has been altered until it is only a caricature of what food should be. This imbalance is the main factor in causing most of the physical and psychiatric disease we must deal with. There will be no relief from the enormous psychosocial, physical, and economic costs of this imbalance until it is corrected, until we return to the whole living diets of our ancestors, or until we adopt the feeding principle and practices of any good zoo. But we know more than did our ancestors 10,000 years ago. We know about nutrient supplements. We should therefore use the best food available and for those with special needs provide the extra quantities required. We should practice the principles of natural or orthomolecular nutrition.

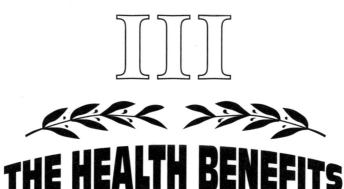

III

THE HEALTH BENEFITS
OF A NATURAL DIET

THE OPTIMUM DIET

ᛦ

INDIVIDUAL ADAPTATION

Most people are convinced that modern high-tech food provides the best in nutrition. This is the message put forward by food industry advertising, by their nutritionists, and by many doctors of the old school. Most doctors know so little about nutrition they will not make any public comment about it, although they are sure that no one needs any vitamin and mineral supplements. This is what they have been taught in medical school by their professors of nutrition, most of whom do not have medical degrees and have had no experience in treating patients whose illness arises from their malnutrition. Overly processed food tastes very good, looks good, satisfies the sensation of hardness or softness in the mouth, and is packaged attractively. Epidemiologists have used measures of health which indicate that our society is healthier than it has ever been, namely the infant mortality rate and the increasing number of people living to retirement age. Some conclude that the high-tech diet has been the main factor in bringing about this apparent high state of good general health. But as I have shown earlier, the high incidence of chronic disease (every second Canadian has one or more chronic diseases) contradicts this claim, as does the ever increasing cost of medical care.

As we have also seen, one of the chief factors in generating

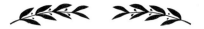

chronic disease is the mismatch between the food to which we have become adapted and the food which we consume. The adaptation developed over evolution has been destroyed by the changes in our foods which have come about so quickly it has been impossible for our digestive apparatus to accommodate them. Most drivers know that they must buy gasoline to operate their cars and oil with which to lubricate it. They know that cars will not work well if diesel oil or water is placed in their gas tank. They know that the type of oil will have to be changed if one drives in very cold weather as opposed to warm weather. If they do not know this they will soon discover it. They know that the cars have been made to run on these products, that these products have been designed to work in the cars, that there is a match between the design of the engine and the type of fuel which is needed. They are not surprised that their car will not work well on the wrong fuel, that it is sick. No amount of tinkering with the car's engine will make those cars well again. This can be achieved only by the use of the right fuel. The same principle applies to our bodies. They have to be fueled with the nutrients which they require to move, keep warm, grow, and maintain good health. We should not be surprised to find that our bodies do not operate properly if given the wrong fuel, if there is a mismatch or maladaptation of diet to body.

All living organisms live within an environment to which they have to adapt. The environment may be relatively constant over enormous periods of time or it may shift very rapidly. Organisms, plants or animals, that cannot adapt to the environments cannot survive. Obviously the rate of adaptation will depend upon the rate at which the environmental changes occur. When the environment changes slowly, there

> *All living organisms live within an environment to which they have to adapt. The environment may be relatively constant over enormous periods of time or it may shift very rapidly. Organisms, plants or animals, that cannot adapt to the environments cannot survive.* **LAW**

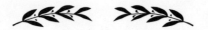

is ample time for the organisms within that environment to adapt and to change. When the environment changes rapidly, there may not be sufficient time and species of living beings may be wiped out very quickly simply because there has not been enough time. Dinosaurs were wiped out over a relatively short period of time by a rapid change in the atmosphere caused by the collision of a large object with earth. This is one of the theories being examined to account for their disappearance after having successfully inhabited this earth for over 100 million years.

Animals may adapt to the change in their environment by changing their habits without needing much if any change in their genetic structure. Genetic changes in animals, excluding insects, tend to be very slow and require long periods of time. Changes in habits may occur very quickly. Modern examples are the invasions of cities in North America by animals such as raccoons, rabbits, deer, and even cougars in Vancouver Island. Rats have survived in the presence of people for thousands of years. These animals have learned to live within environments that would have been intolerable for them a long time ago. Genetic changes occur very slowly, requiring millions of years. Darwin discovered that the pressure to survive created species of animals that favored fitness. Animals best able to survive in the changed environment would be more apt to reproduce and gradually their offspring would become the predominant species. Species that became too rigid in structure, form, or physiology would be less adaptable, and although they could survive, they would not be able to change. Some animals appear to be the same as they were millions of years ago. They have learned how to survive in environments that are fairly stable. Thus evolution, meaning development of more advanced species, does not necessarily go along with survival. Survival also plays a role only during the reproductive periods. For humanity what happens after age 60 is relatively unimportant for the human species in terms of survival of the fittest.

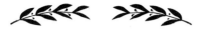

Survival of the fittest applies to the gradual development of better species which increase their proportion of the total gene pool. If our major reproductive period was towards the end of our lives, there would be a much different relationship. But this is a modern phenomenon since more people are alive to retirement whereas throughout evolution the mean age at death was closer to the reproductive period.

The connection between food supply and survival of species is clear. Animals must be provided with food of the type their species has been consuming and to which they have adapted. There is a wide variation in adaptation, ranging from species which appear to have only one major food supply, like the anteater, to species which can consume a wide variety of plants and animals. This has been recognized by animal nutritionists, especially those in charge of modern zoos, but this recognition has been very slow in coming to human nutritionists. Lack of recognition of the need to match our food supply with our inherited needs underlies the health crises of which we hear so much today. Maladaptation is the major factor and must be corrected if ever we are to halt the inevitable increase in chronic disease and bring it back to levels which a proper match of genetics and food supply would ensure.

Everyone knows that every person is unique. Infants know this as soon as they can differentiate their mother from all other mothers. When a child first recognizes a stranger, he or she has already mastered the concept that we are all different. In appearance we are not the same. The best test for this is the interest generated when identical twins walk down the street together. When quintuplets are identical, public curiosity is enormous, for these phenomena violate the principle of individuality. I think the need for individuality was essential for survival. The outer appearance and behavior of any individual is an expression of that person's physiology and biochemistry. It therefore follows that their biochemistry and nutritional needs must also be individual.

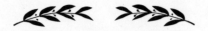

Without individuality there would be no humanity. The individuality of people was necessary for the evolution of our human societies.

We know all about the individuality of finger prints, how even identical twins do not have identical finger prints. Blood types also are unique to individuals as are dental patterns and DNA. Surgeons are not surprised when they try to find the appendix and it is not where it is supposed to be. Sometimes the heart is on the right side. Most organs of the body are not exactly where they are supposed to be, nor are they the same size and shape. Physicians and pharmacologists have known that the optimum doses for drugs can vary enormously between patients, that while there are useful guides for how much to give, many people will need much less and many will need much more. But when it came to the need for optimum nutrition, that knowledge of individuality disappeared, primarily in the medical and nutritional profession. People knew that one "man's meat was another man's poison." They knew that they could eat what others cannot, but the concept was not clearly expressed and was not acted on in developing optimum nutrition.

The manufacture and advertising of high-tech food is based upon the principle that we are all alike, however. Producers of any product will extol the virtues of their product and will not refer to the fact that many people may be allergic or otherwise be made sick by their product and should avoid it. It is unrealistic to expect the manufacturers of high-tech food to refer to the possibility that some may be allergic to their product, but it would be refreshing if they did place the health of their customers somewhere above their idea that this would injure their bottom line. The dairy industry touts its products very highly with support from nutritionists and physicians. But they never discuss in their

> **LAW** *We are unique as individuals and our needs for nutrients vary as do other biochemical and physical attributes.*

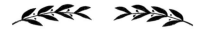

advertisements that many people are made sick by milk.

We are unique as individuals and our needs for nutrients vary as do other biochemical and physical attributes. There will be a narrow range of variation for some nutrients and a wide range of variation for others. Each nutrient will have its own range. This means that most people will have an optimum range which varies about a mean for the whole group, but there will be a much smaller number of people who will need much less and another group who will need very much more.

The optimum amount of nutrients also varies, but we do not have the data for each nutrient on large normal populations. The recommended daily allowances (RDAs) generally cover a very narrow range of need. The developers of these recommended doses assumed that vitamins were needed only in very small doses and added what they considered was an ample safety factor by recommending more than they really thought were needed. However, these doses apply only to healthy people. They, in their definition, excluded people under stress, people who are sick, pregnant women, and nursing women. There are so many exclusions that these RDAs have no value for individuals. They have never been of any value for determining what individuals should be taking. Recently scientists have begun to recognize this, and some have recommended using specific doses for individual diseases. This I have done for many years.

If we constructed a large bell shaped curve showing the range of dosage for any one nutrient along the bottom or the X axis, and plotted the area on the curve where each disease properly fell, we would find that healthy people would be in the area from the lowest doses to somewhat above the mean for the whole group. Patients would be in the high dose area, and the sicker they were, the closer they would lie to the extreme right of the diagram. Thus the average person will get along fairly well with about 3 grams per day of ascorbic

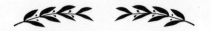

acid. A person with any infection such as the common cold will need perhaps two to three times as much. A person seriously ill with a killing disease such as cancer will require doses ranging from 12 to 40 grams orally and may need an additional 50 to 100 grams given intravenously. Vitamin C represents the very wide variation of optimum doses. Other nutrients have much narrower ranges. Thus for riboflavin there is little evidence to suggest that we have to give more than 100 or 200 mg per day. The water soluble vitamins are very safe because they do not build up in the body. They are easily excreted. Vitamins which are fat soluble can build up and one has to be more cautious about using high doses. But even here the dangers of these vitamins, such as vitamin D-3 and vitamin A, have been grossly exaggerated.

ORTHOMOLECULAR MEDICINE

Dr. Linus Pauling, in his fundamental study of "orthomolecular" nutrition and in his celebrated book *Vitamin C and the Common Cold,* showed how the human body lost its ability during evolution to make certain nutrients. About 20 million years ago man, other primates, the guinea pig, and an Indian fruit-eating bat lost the ability to make vitamin C. The process has not stopped. In my opinion man is going through a process right now when we are losing the ability to make vitamin B-3 from tryptophan. I have suggested in my book *Vitamin B-3 and Schizophrenia: Discovery, Recovery, Controversy* that the schizophrenias represent a group of people who have gone far in this direction. As diets have become high-tech the amount of vitamin B-3 has been lowered, and those people who no longer have the machinery for converting enough tryptophan to the vitamin are becoming sick. I have

> **LAW**
>
> *The new practice of orthomolecular medicine recognizes that most chronic diseases are due to a metabolic fault which is correctable in most patients by good use of nutrition, including the use of vitamin and mineral supplements.*

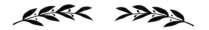

been convinced for a long time that if we were to add 100 mg of niacinamide to our diet for every person, there would be a major decrease in the incidence of schizophrenia and many other diseases such as hyperactivity and learning and behavioral disorders in children.

Dr. Pauling proposed the word "orthomolecular" to describe the use of optimum (often large) doses of molecules naturally present in the body to treat poor health and to promote pure health. The new practice of orthomolecular medicine recognizes that most chronic diseases are due to a metabolic fault which is correctable in most patients by good use of nutrition, including the use of vitamin and mineral supplements. In sharp contrast, drugs are synthetics which are not naturally present in the body and for which the body does not have ready made mechanisms for their destruction and elimination. They are called xenobiotics — that is, foreign molecules. And unlike conventional medicine, orthomolecular medicine also recognizes the principle of individuality in recommending the optimum diet of nutrients for each of us. Orthomolecular medicine requires the application of both these basic principles, individuality and the use of optimum doses (large doses if needed).

WHOLE, ALIVE, FRESH . . .

Just as we were able to describe the problems of the modern high-tech diet with nine adjectives — artifact, dead, stale, monotonous, toxic, abundant, exogenous, synthetic, complex — so we can describe the natural or orthomolecular diet with opposite attributes — whole, alive, fresh, varied, nontoxic, scarce, endogenous, naturally flavored, and simple. The adequacy of these adjectives can be assessed by anyone who has any familiarity with the way animals eat in the wild and the way they are fed in zoos. Natural food is *whole*. Some fish eat other fish swimming less rapidly and they eat them whole. Lions after the kill eat the whole animal provided they

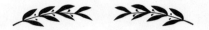

can protect the kill against other predators. A tiger does not cut a steak from its prey and store it either cold or dried or otherwise preserved. Herbivores naturally graze on living vegetable material, although domestic horses and cows are fed grasses which have been cut, dried, and stored.

Whole

Animals that eat their prey will ingest all the available minerals, vitamins, and other food components *whole*. Carnivores often eat the internal organs first and later go after the muscle meats. With plant material there is a tremendous difference nutritionally between the various fractions of that food. Whole wheat is comprised of the germ, the bran, and the white endosperm. The outer coating of the wheat berry or the bran is rich in minerals and vitamins and the richest source of nutrients is the germ. In milling white flour both the bran and the germ are discarded, and by eating the white flour (bread, pastry, pasta) we are depriving ourselves of the most nourishing part of the wheat berry. Nearly 200 years ago it was shown by a French army surgeon that dogs fed on whole meal bread alone were kept alive and healthy, while similar animals fed on white bread quickly sickened and died. Eating whole grain foods provides all the nutrition available in that plant.

Alive

Natural food is *alive*. Even scavenger animals eat meat which has not been stored very long. The main advantage to eating food which is or has been recently alive is that all the nutrients present in that food are available for use. Fresh food, alive or recently alive, has not had time to deteriorate or to develop infection or infestations with organisms and insects that are harmful. Fresh food which has deteriorated loses substantial amounts of vitamins and enzymes. If live food is not always available, the best means of preserving food value is freezing at very low temperatures, and next best

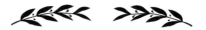

is canning. None of the stored and preserved foods can compare in nutritional quality to the original fresh food. Remember that when animals do store foods, it is food like nuts and seeds which are alive but dormant and which can create new life when given a chance.

Fresh

The third adjective is *fresh*. Fresh and Alive are almost the same since Alive food is necessarily fresh and food which is fresh has been recently alive. But there is a difference. Whole wheat bread which is fresh will be more nutritious than will be the same bread after it has been stored for a long time. With storage there is the problem of contamination with organisms which can destroy the nutrient value of the food and can also cause illness.

Varied

A natural diet is *varied*. By that I mean that since we are omnivores, we can best ensure getting the nutrients we need by consuming a wide variety of foods. The second advantage is that if the foods are varied from meal to meal, from day to day, and from season to season, there is much less danger of developing allergic reactions. If a person is allergic to a food or to several foods, they must be eliminated from the diet often for a period of time lasting from 6 months to a year. Then it may be possible to follow a rotation diet — to follow a schedule where similar families of food are eaten every fourth day or fifth day. A program of eating is developed which spreads the foods over these days. It may then be possible for the person to eat these foods at these intervals without having the usual reactions they were having before.

Modern diets do not follow this principle. Staple foods are consumed daily in large quantities. People will have bread with every meal, meats every day if not in two out of three meals, potatoes every day, and so on. Many individuals eat 50 percent of their calories as sugar. Early man could

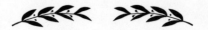

not follow these monotonous diets. Their food supply varied from morning to night, from month to month, and from season to season. They had no way of storing their foods so that they could eat them every day for the whole year.

In meats variety is introduced by eating more than just the muscles. This includes sweetbreads, liver, cartilage, even softer bones. In fish it may include whole fish like sardines. With fruit one can eat from a large variety depending more on the home grown types. The same applies to vegetables. One should consume the edible parts, including leaves, seeds, tubers, roots, and stems where feasible from as many kinds of vegetables as are available. The same applies to grains where one should use all the grains, not just a large number of products made from flour.

Non-toxic

The natural diet is *non-toxic*. It is obvious that our ancestors quickly eliminated those foods which were toxic, probably at first by trial and error. If they ate the food and remained well, this would become part of the diet. They did not have to worry about the addition of chemicals to the food to "enhance" flavor or to preserve it. The foods they ate were non-toxic, except when they tried to store food and it became contaminated with bacteria and their toxins.

Scarce

The food in a natural diet is *scarce*. By scarce I mean in comparison to the abundant food supply available today in high-tech societies. Our ancestors had to adapt to fluctuations in food supply by storing fat as a reserve energy source. During periods when food was abundant, their bodies would store more fat, and when food was scarce or when they were starving, their bodies would draw upon this energy reserve. Women had to bear a double burden when they were pregnant, and for this reason they adapted by storing even more fat before pregnancy and during pregnancy, in order to have enough food to provide milk for their babies. They alternated between having enough food and not having enough, but they did not have to contend with having poor nutritional quality food. Today in high-tech societies there is too much food and there are no periods of starvation or decreased supply. The fat which accumulates when too much is consumed is not taken off by any following period of food reduction or starvation.

Over consumption is less likely with whole meat and fish, fruit and vegetables. It is more of a problem with the grains and nuts and seeds. Sugar is one of the major factors, as are the commercial fats and oils. Natural foods are more bulky, have to be chewed longer and cannot be eaten as quickly so it is less possible to overload the system. Prepared foods from ground and refined grains are usually combined with sugar, fat, and other additives. It is very easy to over-eat bakery goods. Many of my patients with eating disorders have told me that they would buy one dozen doughnuts and that they would be gone before they arrived home, or that they would eat a loaf of bread in one evening, or a pound box of candy in a few hours. Primitive societies did not have a surplus of food. They had to work for their food as well. Modern society does not demand as much calorie expenditure of its people while at the same time providing a huge surplus of attractive artifact foods which taste good and which can easily be eaten very quickly.

Endogenous

Natural food is *endogenous*. Foods before the dawn of agriculture and for thousands of years afterward were locally grown or harvested. Foods today may come from anywhere on the globe. There are both advantages and disadvantages to this. The advantages arise when the imported food is superior in quality to the home grown or endogenous foods. The advantage of home grown food of equal nutritive quality is that there is a better match between the essential fatty

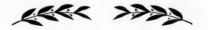

acid composition of the foods in local plants and animals and the fatty acids needed by the consumer of those foods. This is very important in northern and colder climates where the ratio of essential fatty acids to non-essential fats is important in developing cold tolerance. The colder the climate, the more important is it to both plants and animals to have more essential fatty acids. These are more unsaturated and therefore their freezing point is lower. They may be compared to the antifreeze one uses in cars. They are not needed in the tropics but very essential in northern Canada. If a native from Mexico is suddenly transposed to Saskatoon where it is minus 40°F, he will be much more apt to freeze exposed parts of his body — his ears or the rolls of fat around his neck. If the same person moved to Saskatoon in the summer, his body would have time to adjust by laying down more unsaturated fatty acids and he would be much more cold tolerant by the time winter arrived. It is wise to depend as much as possible on endogenous foods but to supplement the diet with exogenous food which is known to be superior in quality.

Naturally Flavored

Natural food is *naturally flavored*. Ancient foods were not overly processed and no synthetic flavors were known. With more sophistication our ancestors began to flavor their foods with herbs. This became much more important when food, which had gone bad, had to be consumed. The herbs were used to cover the awful taste of these stale preparations. Fresh food for most people tastes pretty good, even without the addition of salt and sugar. Many people, however, cannot enjoy the taste of food unless it is saturated with the two substances salt and sugar because that has been so much a part of their diet for so many years.

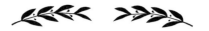

Simple

The natural diet is *simple.* Our ancestors did not have our ability or our desire to compound food preparations. Many modern recipes call for over a dozen different items. In the past the foods were simple and therefore people eating them could know what it was they were eating. If they knew that rabbit meat made them sick, they did not have to worry that some rabbit meat might be present in other food preparations. Today we cannot be sure of the ingredients in food unless we make them ourselves. This is why people who know peanuts will kill them (anaphylactic shock) have died eating food they thought was safe because some person had added peanut oil to the preparation. One has to be very careful of all overly processed foods and to distrust even the labels on many prepared foods.

BALANCED DIET

In the perennial dance of the individual and the environment, time does not go backward. We cannot re-establish the world from which we have evolved. We cannot return to the dietary habitat of our prehistoric ancestors, nor do we need to. It is feasible to process our modern foods and to select from these foods the elements of what we had adapted to. Eventually everything that is done to our food from the farm to our kitchens will have to be treated so as to maximize its nutritional quality. I think we will one day have a public health law which will not permit the sale and distribution of any food preparation unless it is proven that these are as safe and as nourishing as the foods from which they were fashioned. This requires no new knowledge — just the

> *Our food should be processed and selected to fit the description of the diets to which we are adapted. We should be able to describe our foods as almost whole, alive, and fresh and distinguish them from the artifacts that are dead and stale.*

LAW

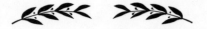

will to do so. It would simply force all the food processors to perform animal feeding tests.

Our food should be processed and selected to fit the description of the diets to which we are adapted. We should be able to describe our foods as almost whole, alive, and fresh and distinguish them from the artifacts that are dead and stale. Visualize a scale or line which ranges from whole at one end (or alive or fresh) to artifact at the other end (or dead or stale). The objective is to move towards the healthy end of the scale as far as possible, knowing that this is an ideal most people won't reach. Nevertheless, it is healthier to be close to the healthy end than it is to be close to the disease end where we are today. Perhaps each item could be rated with a quality item or number starting with 100 and decreasing in value to the pathological end which would be 0. At the zero end life would be barely sustainable with maximum disease, while at the healthy end of the scale life would be sustainable with optimum good health. A quick look at our traditional food groups will reveal how close they come to meeting this natural nutrition standard.

All animal products — meat, fish, eggs, and dairy products — must be as fresh as possible or properly preserved or stored (freeze dried, frozen, or heat dried, which is the less desirable). These foods will have to be cooked unless one is absolutely certain they are free of bacterial or parasitic infection. The only dairy produce which can be considered whole is milk. All the other products are derivative of this. Milk should be fresh and not heat treated if one could be certain it was free of bacterial contamination. Pasteurized milk for most is essential. Cheeses are deliberately contaminated, seeded with organisms which ferment or ripen them. Cheeses cannot be fresh or whole and thus cannot be ideal foods because of the way they are made and stored. Only cottage cheese can meet the fresh criterion; all other cheeses are artifact, dead, and stale, as is ice cream and many other products made from dairy products.

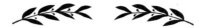

Fresh fruit is alive and almost whole (the seeds are often not consumed). Fruit which has to be stored and shipped is alive and whole to a degree. On storage the fruit will lose a fair amount of its nutritive value, especially the vitamins. This loss is accelerated if the fruit is cut and exposed to air and to light. Frozen fruit is next best to fresh fruit, followed by dried and lastly by preserved fruit. A can of pears is an artifact. The least desirable are the jellies and jams which are mostly sugar flavored by the fruit. Most juices are not wholly healthy foods because they do not meet this criterion.

Fresh vegetables are alive and whole (edible parts only). The quality decreases with processing in factory or in the kitchen in the following order: fast frozen, freeze dried, cooked, and preserved. All edible parts can be used, including roots, tubers, leaves, and stems. On storage vegetables lose vitamins, and when cooked they lose more vitamins and water soluble minerals. They also can become contaminated with bacteria and fungi. Processed fractions from vegetables, such as potato flour, do not meet the criteria since they are artifact, dead, and stale.

Most plant material cannot be digested by people. If consumed, it will be toxic by virtue of this fact and the bulk. Cellulose is indigestible for us but not for fungi and some insects. Straw is indigestible for humans but can be digested by ruminants who have special digestive apparatus for dealing with this. Over the years we have learned which foods are edible. Once we have a tradition about foods it becomes very difficult to change it. For many years tomatoes were considered toxic in the U.S.A. but not in Europe. People began to eat tomatoes in U.S.A. after a public demonstration in front of a court house where one person ate tomatoes. Natural food excludes all the plant and animal material which is inherently toxic or indigestible. The toxic properties of the edible foods arises from the addition of chemicals which have not been proven to be non-toxic in chronic toxicity trials in animals in combination with other

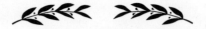

additives or which have not been used by people long enough to have demonstrated its safety.

Whole grains meet the natural standard before they are processed, milled, or ground. They are alive because they can grow. When given the right conditions, they will sprout and produce a whole new plant. They can be consumed whole or may be ground and eaten very soon after that. But once ground they quickly go stale, especially flax which turns rancid very quickly. Bread made from wheat is pretty healthy, even though it is now dead. The nutritive quality for many is enhanced by the cooking, which makes them easier to chew and to digest. The quality decreases quickly with increased refinement in processing.

I do not like the term "balanced" diet because it has been corrupted by dietitians and food processors who use it as a justification for allowing the many degradations in the food they make. For many years apologists for white bread maintained that since no one lived on bread alone, it did not matter if it was deficient in some nutrients. The rest of the nutrients needed to balance the diet, they maintained, would be provided by other food groups than grains. This is not true. If 90 percent of the diet was good, it would not matter too much if 10 percent was corrupted. But where 75 percent of the diet is corrupted, it really does matter. Ideally each food should contain its full share of nutrients required by the person. Whole foods are balanced already by nature. A diet consisting of natural foods is inherently balanced, provided enough variety is introduced. In the animal world monotonous foods are well balanced. An anteater eats a diet of live ants only and the koala bear eats only leaves from a few species of the eucalyptus tree. The term "balanced" should apply only to combinations of natural foods — only to the natural orthomolecular diet.

NUTRIENT SUPPLEMENTS

Optimum adaptation is not perfect adaptation. Perfect adaptation would exist if every cell in the body, every tissue, every organ, and every system were provided with the amount of each nutrient required for optimum growth and function. At the same time all the waste products of metabolism would be removed so as not to interfere with the operation of these cells and tissues. Obviously this is impossible. Optimum adaptation exists when the organism, plant or animal, is in balance with the environment, especially the biochemical environment, so that it can grow, function, and reproduce to perpetuate the species. It does not necessarily mean long life, although long life will accompany optimum adaptation. Since perfect adaptation may not be possible, each cell and each tissue must therefore learn to function adequately with less than optimum provision of nutrients, and to respond quickly to more optimum conditions. The chief means of providing optimum conditions is through the use of nutrient supplements — vitamins and minerals.

Since perfect adaptation may not be possible, each cell and each tissue must therefore learn to function adequately with less than optimum provision of nutrients, and to respond quickly to more optimum conditions. The chief means of providing optimum conditions is through the use of nutrient supplements — vitamins and minerals.

LAW

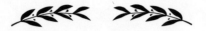

PARADIGM SHIFT

The original impetus to use vitamins therapeutically started in 1955 when I published with my colleagues a research paper showing that niacin (vitamin B-3) lowered cholesterol levels in people. L.J. Machlin, in the *Annals* of the New York Academy of Sciences (1992), credits this report as having started a new age in the medical use of vitamins with our "recognition of health effects beyond prevention of deficiency diseases, new biochemical functions." For the thirty years following our report there was a slow accumulation of papers in the medical literature confirming our findings and expanding them, but very few physicians in the practice of medicine heard about it. They were swayed by the massive advertising in the journals placed by companies promoting their own inferior products for lowering cholesterol. There can be no patent on the use of niacin and therefore it was never promoted by any major drug companies. About eight years ago interest began to increase until the final report of the Coronary Drug Study was published, showing that of all the compounds tested only niacin decreased the death rate (by 11 percent) and increased longevity (by two years). It is the only compound so far tested in long term tests which produced a real decrease. The other compounds decreased mortality a little from cardiovascular disease, but there was a compensating increase in deaths from accidents, suicides, and homicides. This did not occur with niacin. We are now in the rapidly expanding phase of niacin use for lowering cholesterol world wide. It is one of the safest and most effective compounds in lowering cholesterol and increasing HDL.

The second major boost to this concept of using vitamins therapeutically came with our first paper where we showed that vitamin B-3 was therapeutic for schizophrenics. But in sharp contrast to the general acceptance today of this role of vitamins in medicine, psychiatry still has not accepted it and remains where it was 40 years ago.

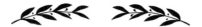

I estimate that the use of large doses of vitamin B-3 is now at the middle of the accelerating phase as more and more information is disseminated in the medical and popular literature. Interest has also spread to the other vitamins, particularly the antioxidant vitamins such as vitamin E, vitamin C, and beta carotene — and to the antioxidant minerals such as selenium. Other diseases being examined where therapeutic doses of vitamins can be used are cancer, AIDS, mental disease, cardiovascular disease, senility. Within about ten years the maturation phase will have been reached and even medical schools will be teaching their students all about the therapeutic use of vitamins — about orthomolecular medicine.

The history of the use of food and vitamins for medicinal purposes has been divided into five ages by Dr. L.J. Machlin. The first period ranges from about 1500 B.C. to 1900. Foods were used empirically to heal certain diseases. The second period ranges from 1880 to 1900. During this period deficiency diseases were produced in animals, and the vitamin hypothesis was developed. The third period ranges from 1900 to 1930. During this phase the vitamins were discovered, isolated, their structure determined, and their synthesis established. The fourth period begins about 1930 when biochemical functions of the body were studied, dietary requirements were introduced, and commercial production of vitamins became prominent. We are now into the fifth period which began in 1955 and is characterized by the recognition of therapeutic health effects beyond prevention of deficiency disease.

From 1880 to 1955, vitamins were limited in their application to the prevention of deficiency diseases such as beri beri and pellagra. During this vitamin-as-prevention era, it was believed that the only role of vitamins was to prevent vitamin deficiency diseases, and they were needed in small amounts. This made sense since vitamins were catalysts of reactions in the body and catalysts are known to be needed

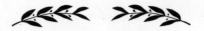

only in small amounts as they are used over and over. Any dose above these small preventive doses was undesirable, wasteful, bad medical practice, and, to some, even criminal. Physicians have lost their medical license because of the unsubstantiated charges that they were prescribing large doses of vitamins that harmed their patients. Some hospitals still do not permit the use of intravenous ascorbic acid. These 'principles' make up the preventative vitamin or vitamin deficiency paradigm. They are still adhered to very vigorously by many dietitians, nutritionists, and physicians.

The old paradigm led to the creation of RDAs (recommended daily allowances) which have been like the holy writ for many years in spite of the fact they were designed to provide guidelines for only the healthy part of the population. They are of no value to individuals who are not average — not of value to 50 percent of the total population. Orthomolecular therapists have consistently argued against their use and have ignored them in their practices. Recently, Professor David Mark Hegsted, appointed to Harvard's New England Regional Primate Research Center in Southborough, Massachussets, recommended the RDAs be abolished, arguing that the system is unworkable because it was based on estimates using healthy young males — the group least likely in the population to have nutritional deficiencies. Dr. J. Blumberg, Professor of Nutrition at Tufts University, argues that "the RDA committee is locked into the old paradigm of nutrition — how much is needed to prevent deficiency disease. It has not shifted gears to where medicine is today."

In the middle 1930s just after it was recognized that niacin cured pellagra, the early pellagrologists found, I am certain to their great surprise, that the small doses of vitamin B-3 which prevented pellagra and which cured early (acute) pellagra did not help patients who had chronic pellagra. They required 600 mg per day, a huge quantity, compared to the tiny dose of less than 20 mg needed to prevent pellagra. This proved that the optimum dose even to prevent pellagra from

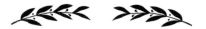

recurring ranged from 20 to 600 mg daily. Chronic pellagra changed body chemistry (in humans and dogs) so that the small doses effective as a preventative measure were no longer adequate. Much larger amounts were needed, for they had developed a dependency on vitamin B-3. A deficiency is present when the diet is so bad that even the small preventive doses are not provided. A dependency is present when the needs of the body are so great that even the best diet cannot provide the right amount. The preventative vitamin paradigm does not recognize this therapeutic vitamin "law."

> *A dependency is present when the needs of the body are so great that even the best diet cannot provide the right amount. The preventative vitamin paradigm does not recognize this therapeutic vitamin "law."*   **LAW**

As such, the preventive vitamin paradigm as been very harmful to nutritional research. It inhibited the investigations of the therapeutic use of vitamins for at least 30 years. It is still harmful because it still has the medical school departments of nutrition in its sway. It is correct only for the very few classical deficiency diseases and is totally incorrect for the rest of medicine.

Our research published in 1955 proposed the therapeutic use of vitamins in large doses. The therapeutic vitamin paradigm is based on the following four observations. (1) We are all different and have different nutrient requirements. (2) Optimum amounts of vitamins are needed which range from smaller doses necessary to prevent deficiency disease to much larger doses to treat vitamin dependent conditions — conditions like elevated cholesterol levels and too low levels of high density lipoprotein cholesterol. (3) The following variables determine the optimum need: age, sex, physical stress including pregnancy, psychological stress, lactation, diseases (whether acute or chronic), use of xenobiotic drugs. Thus there can never be one useful Optimal Daily Dose (ODD) schedule for everyone. There must be an Optimal Recommended Dose

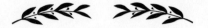

(ORD) specific for each condition and for each disease. (4) Vitamins can be taken safely for a life time.

The therapeutic vitamin paradigm opens up the use of vitamins for optimum health to everyone. In sharp contrast to drugs, which are very toxic and must be carefully controlled by trained professionals, vitamins are so safe they can be experimented with by any person secure in the knowledge that they are as safe as are any of the over-the counter medications readily available today. People can become their own therapists. Experimentation will not do them any harm, provided they have have taken a little time to examine the vitamin literature. With drugs too little is much safer than too much, but with vitamins a little more is much safer than too little if one wishes to obtain optimum health. If more than is needed is taken, there is no harm because the extra amount is not stored and is readily eliminated. There are very few exceptions. Thus one can try to find the optimum by taking increasing doses until it is reached. And if that dose is exceeded, the body can readily deal with it. If too little is taken, the desired therapeutic effect will not be obtained. The difference between optimum and less effective doses can be narrow. I have seen schizophrenic patients who did not respond to 3 grams per day of niacin, but when this was doubled, they began to improve very quickly. The same principle does not apply to minerals and may not apply to amino acids, even though they also have a wide tolerance range.

> **LAW**
>
> *The therapeutic vitamin paradigm opens up the use of vitamins for optimum health to everyone. In sharp contrast to drugs, which are very toxic and must be carefully controlled by trained professionals, vitamins are so safe they can be experimented with by any person secure in the knowledge that they are as safe as are any of the over-the-counter medications readily available today. People can become their own therapists.*

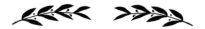

The year 1992 was a watershed year in public attitudes toward vitamin therapy, marking a great turn around in medical interest in the use of vitamins for therapy, using doses much larger than ever before recommended or accepted. It was inevitable but pleasant at last to see. The lay press, which had for years been toeing the party line about nutrients and the RDAs, suddenly began to publish reports about the remarkable new therapeutic properties of the vitamins. Since the media feel free, at last, to publish this information, it is clear they are no longer afraid of the censure of the old medical establishment and that the profession has become interested enough that it no longer objects as vigorously as it did in the past. There are a few fossilized physicians who are still living in the early twentieth century but they are rapidly fading from the scene.

One of the first signs of this new age of vitamin therapy was an article published in *The New York Times*, March 10, 1992 under the headline "Vitamins Win Support as Potent Agents of Health." *The New York Times* had not been as enthusiastic a decade earlier when the paper commissioned a freelance reporter to attend a meeting of the Huxley Institute of Biosocial Research in New York. I was then president of HIBS. This meeting was given greetings by Mayor Koch. After the two-day meeting, the reporter approached me for an interview, which he prefaced by telling me that he had expected to find a bunch of strange people and kooks at this meeting. Instead he found a medical group of the highest order and sobriety reporting on their findings. I initially refused to spend any time with him when he told me he was from the *Times*, suspecting they would not publish anything favorable about our work. He then assured me that he had never had an article rejected by his editors. With that assurance I spent about six hours with him outlining the work, answering all his questions. The report never appeared. There is no doubt he wrote a favorable report but this was

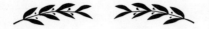

not something the *Times* wanted since they were still under the sway of the medical 'profession.'

Time Magazine, April 6, 1992, was next with their cover story "The Real Power of Vitamins," subtitled "New Research Shows They May Help Fight Cancer, Heart Disease and the Ravages of Aging." While the U.S. Food and Drug Administration (FDA) disputed nutrient health claims, Dr. Walter Willett of the Harvard School of Health said, "at this time I say don't take megadoses, but I'm not ruling out that in two or three years we might change our mind." The *Time* report concluded: "But stay tuned. Vitamins promise to continue to unfold as one of the great and hopeful health stories of our day." *The Medical Post*, April 23, 1992, reported that vitamin C may lower heart disease risk, and on May 8, 1992 the *New York Times* reported, "Vitamin C Linked to Heart Benefit: It May Also Help Prevent an Early Death from Other Disease." *Newsweek* finally joined ranks May 8, 1992 with their story "Live Longer With Vitamin C." *The Harvard Health Letter, Johns Hopkins Medical Letter*, and the *Diet-Heart Newsletter* have reported with similar stories. Finally, the U.S. National Institutes of Health has created a new Office of Alternative Medicine which will explore various alternative practices. I hope the study of vitamins will be included in their mandate — unless they now consider megavitamin therapy as mainstream medicine.

The medical profession has been alerted to this new age by the *New England Journal of Medicine* in a 1993 article which reported that in 1990 more Americans consulted alternative practitioners than all U.S. primary care physicians, 425 million visits versus 388 million. The social demographic group who consulted these alternative practitioners were non-black, ranging in age from 25 to 49 years, with relatively more education and higher incomes. They consulted them for chronic conditions. Twelve percent of this group sought megavitamin therapy — 51 million visits were devoted to megavitamin therapy. The authors advised the profession should ascertain from

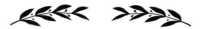

their patients information about their use of alternative therapies. I do not think this will be much help since most patients who have consulted me are not willing to discuss it with their practitioners because of the negative reactions they have had in the past. The article concluded that "medical schools should include information about unconventional therapies and the clinical social sciences (anthropology and sociology) in their curriculums. The newly established National Institutes of Health Office for the Study of Unconventional Medical Practices should help promote scholarly research and education in this area."

(It would also help if the *New England Journal of Medicine* would relax its censorship of reports dealing with megavitamin therapy. Several years ago they absolutely refused to publish a rebuttal by Linus Pauling of an article on cancer and vitamin C which was faulty, badly done, and little deserving of the publicity it generated.)

British and Canadian doctors are also facing growing pressure from alternative medicine, as C. Gray in the *Canadian Medical Association Journal* writes: "It is impossible to ignore the growing acceptance of alternative medicine in today's Britain." She predicts that in Canada the future promises a "similar change. Alternative medicine is beginning to find a ready and healthy market. And our doctors as a group are feeling unloved and unrewarded." Vitamin therapy (megavitamin) is well on the way to sweeping the field.

NUTRIENT DEPENDENCY

Most nutrients can be obtained from the natural diet. Before launching into a nutrient supplement regimen, be sure to

---

One cannot compensate for a poor diet by taking huge quantities of supplements. They are to be taken after the diet has been made as good as possible and if thereafter the state of health desired has not been reached.

LAW

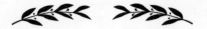

read the chapter on "The Nutrient Content of Common Foods" later in this book. It is important to know that supplements, no matter how valuable, do not replace food. One cannot compensate for a poor diet by taking huge quantities of supplements. They are to be taken after the diet has been made as good as possible and if thereafter the state of health desired has not been reached.

You will have to find out for yourself which vitamin and other nutrients you should take as a supplement and how much from the information given for each nutrient. The nutrients I will not describe have not been used therapeutically, but it is likely that in time every nutrient will be found to be essential in large amounts for some disease. I am convinced that there are some common diseases which are nutrient dependent, that there are some very rare diseases which are not treated well today which are dependent on one or more nutrients. Thus, I think Huntingtons Disease is a double dependency on vitamin E and vitamin B-3.

Indeed, for every nutrient there are individuals who are dependent upon it, and if it is not provided they will suffer a disease or a syndrome. This disease will not be adequately treated until this nutrient is discovered and it is given in optimum quantities. There will be fewer individuals who will be dependent upon two nutrients, and even fewer who will be dependent upon three or more. The greater the number of dependencies the less likely that individual will survive beyond infancy.

After having restored the foods and nutrition to what we have adapted to as closely as possible, it is then necessary to determine whether supplements are needed. One day this will be done by careful laboratory tests, but these are still in the experimental stages and are not readily available.

> **LAW**
>
> *Indeed, for every nutrient there are individuals who are dependent upon it, and if it is not provided they will suffer a disease or a syndrome.*

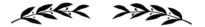

Furthermore they are expensive. The easiest and most accurate way is to use oneself as the test organism, proceeding by trial and error. The trials are simple and the errors are minimal. There is no better method. If you wanted to be even more precise, you could have the pharmacist make up the vitamin to be tested and a matching set of pills which are identical in everything except they would contain an inert substance. They could be coded so that you would not know which was which. Then one set of pills would be taken, say for two months, and after that the other. Notes would be kept of any changes in health to determine which is the superior product. If this could not be determined, it would mean that this particular vitamin or nutrient is not needed. This would be a so-called double blind controlled experiment with a series of one.

The starting dose must be enough to produce the desired effect. A dose too small would not be helpful. Once it has been found that the nutrient has had an appreciable effect, you could then increase the dose to determine if more would improve health even more. The dose range will be indicated for each nutrient. Side effects should be recorded. With an increase in dose these side effects would be more pronounced. You would have to be sure that the side effects are coming from the active nutrient and not from some other ingredient in the composition. For example, many are allergic to yeast, and if the nutrient is yeast based, there will be side effects from the yeast, wrongfully ascribed to the nutrient.

My daughter, a dietitian nutritionist, is not as hopeful as I am that people can be persuaded to alter their diets. She may well be right. For these people the less than ideal program will be to take the supplements anyway since they will provide some of the nutrients that are missing from their diet. It is simpler to swallow pills than it is to change cooking and eating habits. If this is the only concession some people will make to change, then at least they should increase their intake of all the water soluble vitamins.

VITAMIN C

꧁

Very few people knew about vitamin C until Professor Linus Pauling issued his first book on *Vitamin C and the Common Cold* in 1970. There was a marked increase in sales of vitamin C following that report. This was so disturbing to the medical community they began a major effort to discredit Dr. Pauling, even to the point of calling him senile, trying to debunk his conclusion that vitamin C would be preventive *and* therapeutic for the common cold and for other conditions. A main complaint was that Dr. Pauling, awarded Nobel Prizes for Biochemistry and Peace, was not a medical doctor and therefore should not be commenting on medical matters. One physician in Australia tried to link the resulting increased use of vitamin C to an equally dramatic rise in the incidence of kidney stones. He did not mention that the increase in kidney stones had begun long before Dr. Pauling's book appeared and that after it appeared the incidence did not rise any further. A letter of rebuttal that I submitted to the journal which carried this report was rejected. Since then there has been a massive effort on the part of many doctors, dietitians, professors of biochemistry, and others to educate people against taking vitamin supplements because the average diet provided all that was needed. They linked vitamin C to every possible toxicity. Yet the public has its own way of dealing with medical ideas. It goes by how it feels. When a patient finds that he gets fewer colds

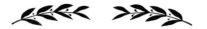

after taking vitamin C, no amount of rhetoric will persuade him that his own convictions are unscientific. In any event the tide has turned and the once shrill voices against vitamin C have calmed down as more physicians have entered the megavitamin field. As an illustration of the increased demand, the price of ascorbic acid has gone up $3.75 per kilogram in the past year. The supply has not kept up with demand. The manufacturers will have to build new plants to match the increased demand.

In spite of intense opposition, Linus Pauling's conclusion that vitamin C was helpful in decreasing the frequency and ravages of the common cold has won the day. Many scientific studies have shown that vitamin C consistently decreases the duration of cold episodes and the severity of symptoms; and if all these investigators had followed the advice given by Dr. R. Cathcart, that optimum doses should be used, there would have been a decrease in frequency of colds as well. This has been amply confirmed by the patients who have been taking the vitamin in higher doses and who report that the frequency of their colds has been greatly decreased, compared to the number of colds their close relatives are still getting. As Dr. Pauling has said, "Since I began writing in this field, I've had the support of scientists. They say that I've been right so often that I'm probably right here too. It's the medical community that has been blind. Rene Dubois, who discovered the first antibiotics, said that he was always working in the mainstream of science, but I was 20 years ahead of everyone else. I myself don't consider myself a maverick in science. I'm just ahead of it."

Every human suffers from subclinical scurvy, from a deficiency of vitamin C or ascorbic acid. We cannot make any in our bodies, and the amount present in even the best possible diet will not provide more than 100 mg per day. This amount is totally inadequate for optimum health. There is no need to ask the question, do I need any vitamin C? The only question is how much is needed. There are many clues in nature. Of

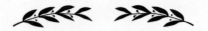

these the best is the amount of vitamin C which animals make in their body normally and also under severe stress. They are able to convert glucose into vitamin C. They make much more than we take in from our food. Thus a goat, weighing about as much as a man, will make 14 grams of vitamin C per day. Apparently all animals that make vitamin C make about the same amount per kilogram of body weight. Since we lost the capability of making vitamin C about 20 million years ago, our bodies have had to adapt to chronic deficiency after we moved away from a natural diet to a food supply that did not provide adequate amounts. We are still paying the price of this dietary change, but we no longer have to since synthetic ascorbic acid is very inexpensive. Every person should take ample quantities to replace what nature took away from us. Although we are not as sick as if we had scurvy, this is small consolation since scurvy is a terminal disease. I do not think we should be content with being just some distance away from death.

Because of our modern high-tech diet, the symptoms of scurvy are still alive and well. Several doctors have documented cases in the United States among men ranging in age from 35 to 61 who suffered painful edema on the legs, red spots on their arms, abdomen, and legs as well as large purple discolorations on the lower limbs. They ate frequently in restaurants, avoided fruits and vegetables. Given ascorbic acid they responded in a few days. Dr. Linus Pauling and Dr. Rath have shown that the body increases its production of lipoprotein cholesterol (a) in an attempt to overcome some of the symptoms of scurvy. A major problem with scurvy is that the blood vessels can no longer retain their integrity and fluid leaks from them, into the skin, into the tissues. The lipoprotein (a) present in the blood plugs small leaks which develop and decreases the leakage of fluid from the vessels. But if too much is made — and this could be a *too* successful attempt to prevent fluid loss — the extra lipoprotein(a) is deposited in the vessel wall and initiates arteriosclerosis. This is one of the main factors responsible for cardiovascular disease,

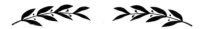

including strokes and coronary disease. There are probably other mechanisms which have developed over the past 20 million years to try and overcome the problems generated by the lack of ascorbic acid.

CHIEF ANTIOXIDANT

Vitamin C is therefore needed by everyone, not only to prevent diseases like scurvy but also to insure optimum health of the whole body. And in the presence of any pathology or stress, the amount needed increases very rapidly. It has been found that the more serious the condition the more vitamin C is needed. A good indicator of this is the ratio of ascorbic acid in its original reduced state to the amount of oxidized vitamin C, dehydroascorbic acid. Normally less than 5 percent of the total vitamin C in the body is in the oxidized state so that the ratio is better or higher than 20:1. However, when the individual is close to death almost all the vitamin C is in the oxidized state and the ratio is very small. For other diseases the amount of oxidized vitamin C decreases. In people who are very sick and begin to recover the amount of oxidized vitamin goes down quickly. It is apparent that the vitamin C must be in the reduced state since only then can it function as an antioxidant. The best way to ensure that the ratio is very low is to take ample quantities of the vitamin.

> *Vitamin C is therefore needed by everyone, not only to prevent diseases like scurvy but also to insure optimum health of the whole body. And in the presence of any pathology or stress, the amount needed increases very rapidly.*
>
> **LAW**

Vitamin C is indeed our chief antioxidant. We live in an atmosphere which contains about 20 percent oxygen. This is used in respiration to create energy. But excessive oxidation will be very harmful. Free radicals are formed which are very active and can damage cells and tissues. A free radical can pull another electron from another molecule and convert

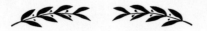

that into another free radical. This chain reaction will continue until the electron reacts with another electron, or is deactivated by an antioxidant, a scavenger, or an enzyme. The body has developed a system of antioxidants to protect itself against excessive oxidation. In the same way a potato will not turn brown until it is pealed and exposed to air. The brown pigment formed is the result of excessive oxidation in a tissue not protected by antioxidants. Vitamin C is the main water soluble antioxidant, but the body's defense system also includes other nutrients that work in conjunction with vitamin C, including antioxidant enzymes, superoxide dismutase (SOD), catalase, glutathione peroxidase, vitamin E, beta carotene, non-enzymatic scavengers, uric acid, glutathione, and thiols in proteins.

These substances work together both within the cell and in the fluids outside the cells. They also reinforce each others activity: for example, vitamin E spares vitamin C. Vitamin C works mainly in the water medium, while vitamin E works primarily in the fat medium and on cell membranes.

Free radicals are involved an a large number of processes in the body, including cancer, aging, Parkinson's disease, cardiovascular disease, cataracts, arthritis, and diabetes. By controlling these reactions antioxidants have a therapeutic role in all these conditions.

OPTIMUM DOSAGE

The maximum recommended oral dose of vitamin C is 75 grams each day, but very few can tolerate this extremely high dose because it exceeds the laxative dose. While the majority of people take under 12 grams per day, it is best to think in terms of the optimum tolerable dose. Each person can determine this for themselves. When more vitamin C is taken than that individual can absorb from the gastrointestinal tract, it causes increased formation of gas and the bowel contents become very fluid. If the dose greatly exceeds this level,

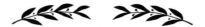

diarrhea will develop. The ideal dose has optimum functions in the body without causing any effect on the bowel except to help regulate it. It is a very good laxative. Since at least one third of the population over 65 is constipated, it would seem to me to be wise for all elderly people to control this problem not only by consuming enough fiber but also by taking enough vitamin C. This is done by starting with doses of 3 to 6 grams each day and gradually increasing it until the sublaxative dose is reached. Then the dose is decreased to just below this level. If the laxative level is 20 grams, the optimum oral level will be around 18 grams. Dr. R. Cathcart discovered that the more the body needs the vitamin, the more it can tolerate. I have observed the same, as have almost all orthomolecular physicians. My optimum dose has ranged between 30 and 3 grams daily depending on my state of health. If a lot more is needed, it is possible to train the body to accept more. Some AIDS cases in Australia have been trained to take 200 grams daily. If the higher doses cannot be reached, it may be necessary to take intravenous vitamin C. When given in IV drip, up to 200 grams can be given over several hours without any gastrointestinal effect.

Vitamin C is a weak organic acid, comparable to lemon juice. Compared to the strong acid present in the stomach, the addition of any amount of ascorbic acid makes a minor contribution to the stomach fluid acidity. Still, a number of people do not like the sour taste. For this reason it is fortunate that the salts of ascorbic acid are available. They are sodium ascorbate, potassium ascorbate, calcium ascorbate, etc. A few preparations on the market contain a variety of these salts of vitamin C. They are called mineral ascorbates. They do represent an improvement over the straight ascorbic acid which is never present in nature as the pure acid, as it is in tablets, but is associated with other nutrients. One such preparation I have been using for several years is Supergram Plus, non-acidic vitamin C. It contains calcium, magnesium, zinc, manganese, molybdenum, and chromium ascorbates,

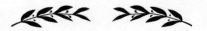

but most of the vitamin C there is sodium ascorbate. It is a good preparation containing other essential nutrients as well. The mineral ascorbates are more tolerable for many and are equivalent to taking the pure vitamin C (hydrogen ascorbate). A very small number of people, fewer than 20 seen over the past 30 years, cannot tolerate any amount of vitamin C. They have developed an allergy or idiosyncrasy to either the synthetic vitamin C or to some of the other ingredients of the preparations. They might try preparations made from other sugar sources. The common vitamin C is made from corn syrup. It is preferable to take the vitamin several times per day to decrease the amount lost in the urine.

Opponents of the use of vitamin C claim that taking more than a few milligrams per day is useless since the vitamin C is excreted into the urine. They cynically refer to urine rich in vitamin C. This, of course, is a foolish argument that only those ignorant of how vitamin C is absorbed and excreted could use. They ignore the fact that in most cases enough of any therapeutic compound must be given before it can be therapeutic and that this sometimes means allowing a major part to appear in the urine. If a person is given 50 grams per day of penicillin to save his life, most of that also appears in the urine. With vitamin C it has been shown that the more that is taken into the body, the greater is the amount retained and used by the body. In our early research we found we could inject chronic schizophrenics with 90 grams of vitamin C and could find none in the urine. If the dose is 1 gram, a fraction of that will be retained. If the dose is 10 grams, many grams will be excreted but many grams will also be retained. To increase the retention, the dose must be increased.

REMARKABLY SAFE

Every time an organism interacts with the environment two possibilities have to be evaluated. Is the interaction beneficial

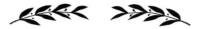

or is it harmful? Given an answer to these questions, then we need to ask, how can one determine the risk involved? How can one balance the potential benefit against the potential harm? There is always a risk-benefit ratio, even in crossing the street. Here the gain is that we are getting close to our goal, the risk is that we will be hit by a car. Activities may be risk free and enormously beneficial — for example, eating good food to which one has been adapted. On the other hand, the potential benefit may be minimal and the risk enormous — for example, in smoking and drinking alcohol or imbibing other poisons. The same applies to all medicines and of course to all nutrients. And it applies also all to the interaction between doctors and their patients.

Even the psychosocial exchanges can profoundly influence a patient's welfare and life expectancy. Telling a patient that he has a killer disease, such as AIDS or cancer, will have a profound influence on that patient depending upon the way that information is given. If the information is given honestly but in a positive way, the patient will be shocked but not nearly as much as he would be if given the same information in a negative way. I have seen hundreds of cancer patients who were told by their oncologist that they had cancer and that they would die in a given time. In one case a patient was told she would be dead in one week and therefore there was no point in giving her a follow-up appointment. In fact, on a vitamin program she lived another 30 months. If the approach is that there is nothing more to be done, the gain to that patient is low and the harm is great — the ratio of gain over risk is too low. If the patient is advised that she has a serious illness which is life threatening but that more can be done — that the physician will be willing to work with that patient and that the chances are better than they might think — then the gain is greater and the harm is less, thus increasing the ratio of good over evil. Every interaction between physician and patient must be evaluated in this way. It applies as well to the medication that is prescribed.

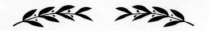

In pharmacology, in the study of drugs, each drug is assessed for its therapeutic effect and for its toxicity. This is mandatory. The drug will not be released for general patient use unless the government agencies are convinced that the drugs are effective and relatively safe. These studies are done by feeding the drugs first to a variety of animals for a long enough period of time. Since animals used in the laboratory are short lived, they are on the drugs for a substantial proportion of their life span. The animals are examined for any pathological changes in their organs, for the effect the drugs have on growth rate, on their ability to reproduce, and of course for the LD_{50}. This is a measure of the ability of drugs to kill. If given over a certain amount of time a dose kills 50 percent of the population of animals, the dose which will do so is called the LD_{50}.

Every physician who has studied the medical literature and has used ascorbic acid knows that it is safe. I can best describe how safe it is by quoting from a report prepared by Dr. John Marks, Fellow, Tutor and Director of Medical Studies, Girton College, Cambridge: "This is a vitamin that has been consistently administered in high dosages for very prolonged periods. Quantities in excess of 1 gram are being ingested by many people as a prophylactic against the common cold, in various cancers, in the detoxification of drug addicts, in schizophrenias, for wound healing and for the prevention of the formation of nitrosamines in the stomach. Some critics of high dose vitamin C administration have alleged that the substance causes kidney stones through the increased excretion of oxalate: interference with vitamin B-12 metabolism; rebound scurvy upon sudden cessation of therapy; excessive iron absorption and a mutagenic effect.

"An extensive and very thorough analysis of the data during the past years has disproved all the serious allegations. Some patients, particularly in the early days of high-dose administration, do experience a laxative effect. Even this mild and harmless adverse effect is not found consistently."

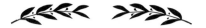

In my opinion the potential danger from ascorbic acid producing kidney stones is grossly exaggerated. There is a known frequency of kidney stone episodes among the general population; it is much less than expected among ascorbic acid users. Dr. R. Cathcart, who has had experience with more patients on ascorbic acid than any other physician, told me that, in his practice, he saw very few cases. The main factor in kidney stones formation appears instead to be a deficiency of magnesium. The false idea that ascorbic acid creates kidney stones arose through the effort of one physician, Dr. V. Herbert. In a letter to the *Canadian Medical Association Journal*, I tried to correct this myth, pointing out that the original methods used for measuring oxalate were faulty and that when an accurate method was used there was no increase. Yet the myth that ascorbic acid may cause kidney stones persists. My criticism of the present oxalate studies are that they are not long term studies. For example, in one study kidney stone patients were given one dose of vitamin C, up to 2 grams of ascorbic acid, on the second or third day post-operative after lithotripsy (removing kidney stones). They still had nephrostomy tubes in. With the 2 grams dose, the doctors conducting the study found an increase of oxalate from 6 mg before to 13 mg afterward. On the basis of this flimsy study they concluded that "patients with a history of stone disease or those who have decreased renal function should certainly be discouraged from taking more than the recommended daily allowance of vitamin C." I think that doctors with this type of evidence should be discouraged from publishing them. On the basis of one small study on patients fresh out of surgery with a tube still in their body (severe stress) and with a minor increase in oxalate they come to this sweeping conclusion. They do not refer to their finding that the increase in oxalate was greatest with the 1 gram dose and was the same for the 500 mg and for the 2 gram doses. There is certainly no consistent dose response curve. It is indeed possible that ascorbic acid helped

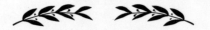

clear oxalates from these patients which had accumulated before they had their stones crushed and removed. Yet this paper will receive massive citations from the critics of ascorbic acid. No study will be valid until it is done on patients who are under normal stress and who have taken ascorbic acid for long periods of time.

I have been taking ascorbic acid in doses ranging from 3 to 30 grams per day, usually below 10 grams, for the past 35 years. I have none of the potential side effects described by the cynical critics of the use of ascorbic acid. I believe I represent almost all of the subjects who take this vitamin. It is remarkably safe.

TREATMENT FOR AGING, ITP, CANCER

Several years ago Linus Pauling stated in his book *How To Live Longer and Feel Better* that people taking ascorbic acid would live longer. All the information we have about ascorbic acid led to this conclusion. But the final test is the practical one — does it work? In fact it does. Dr. James Enstrom, School of Public Health, University of California at Los Angeles, analyzed a ten year study of 11,348 people, aged 25 to 74. Men who consumed at least 300 mg of ascorbic acid suffered 41 percent fewer deaths during that period compared with men who took only 50 mg in their food. They lived on the average six years longer. For women the results were not as striking. This amount of ascorbic acid cannot be obtained from the diet alone and shows that supplements are essential. Had they used gram doses daily, I think the results would have been more striking.

Dr. A.G. Brox and his colleagues at McGill University in Montreal found that ascorbic acid, given 2 grams daily, successfully treated seven out of 11 patients with idiopathic thrombocytopenic purpura (ITP). They had all been sick more than two months and had not responded to adrenocorticosteroids. Three had had splenectomies. Four had

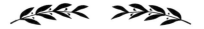

failed additional treatment, including the current usual treatments. I have one patient now with ITP on ascorbic acid who has been well over five years but only as long as she remains on her ascorbic acid. If she discontinues, her platelet count begins to sink within a few weeks.

In 1990, the National Cancer Institute co-sponsored a meeting on Ascorbic Acid and Cancer. Thirty-three presenters, including Linus Pauling, outlined the current state of research connecting vitamin C and cancer. Based upon these abstracts it is clear ascorbic acid must be a major component in the treatment of cancer for the following reasons. It protects plasma lipids against peroxidation. Higher vitamin C levels in the blood provided the most protection. Since both chemotherapy and radiation increase peroxidation, vitamin C decreases the toxicity of these treatments for normal tissue. In vitro ascorbic acid protects cells against transformation by methyl cholenthrene and against Rous sarcoma virus. In hairless mice it decreased the incidence and delayed the onset of malignant lesions when exposed to ultraviolet light. It also decreased incidence of spontaneous mammary tumors in mice. Other workers reported similar protective effects of ascorbic acid on animals. A review of the literature showed that in 33 out of 46 studies vitamin C was protective, decreasing incidence and mortality. Individuals in the top one-quarter vitamin levels had only 50 percent of the cancer risk of those in the lowest quarter. The final conclusion was that ascorbic acid was an important part of any cancer treatment.

Ewan Cameron and Linus Pauling's conclusion in their book *Cancer and Vitamin C* that ascorbic acid increased the survival of patients with terminal cancer first aroused my interest. Subsequently, I began to give cancer patients a comprehensive orthomolecular program which included ascorbic acid, 12 or more grams daily, plus a large number of other nutrients, including vitamin B-3, beta carotene, selenium, and in some cases vitamin E. My patients were also concerned, anxious, or depressed, and were given psychiatric

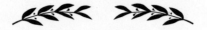

treatment, including medication for this if required. My treatment program proved to be very successful to the point where many doctors began referring their cancer patients to me in substantial number. The first case was a woman with cancer of the pancreas, after a by-pass operation. On this vitamin program she recovered and is still well today, 15 years later. She began to tell all her friends and others about her own recovery and gradually the number of referrals began to increase. When I had seen 134 patients I reviewed their state and sent the information to Dr. Linus Pauling for analysis. He had just developed a new elegant way for examining the outcome of cohort studies. We first published the results in the *Journal of Orthomolecular Medicine*; an expanded study appears in the 1993 edition of Cameron and Pauling's *Cancer and Vitamin C*; and my final work is published in my own book, *Vitamin C and Cancer: Discovery, Recovery, Controversy.*

Of the 134 cases studied, there were 33 patients who did not follow the treatment regimen and 101 similar patients who did. We used the Hardin Jones biostatistical analyses of mortality for cohorts or groups of cancer patients, developed by Dr. Pauling. This method applies to the problem of evaluating mean survival time for a cohort with a few survivors at the termination of the study, and for a cohort with many survivors at the termination of the study. There were three cohorts: (1) The pseudo control group of 33 who did not follow the treatment protocol; they survived 5.7 months. This group included all the cancer cases. (2) The cohort of 40 patients with cancer of the breast, ovary, uterus, cervix, and fallopian tubes. There were 22 survivors. Mean survival time was estimated to be 99 months. (3) The remaining cohort of 61 patients with the other cancers. There were 29 survivors; mean estimated survival time was 67 months. We concluded that 80 percent of the patients who followed my orthomolecular nutritional regimen had a probable survival time 21 times that of the controls for cohort two and 13 times that of

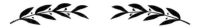

the controls for cohort 3, or for all patients 16 times that of the controls. The mean survival of patients from each group who did not survive was about ten months or about twice as high as it was for those who did not follow the program. The mean survival of the controls, 5.7 months, is about what is observed for ambulatory patients who have reached or are close to the terminal stage of cancer with 85 percent having received potentially curative or palliative conventional therapy.

We concluded that "the much longer mean survival time of 81 of the similar patients who followed the regimen, 92 months, must surely be attributed to this regimen." We also said that "on the basis of these results and of those reported by Cameron and his collaborators we strongly recommended that patients with cancer follow the regimen described in this paper, as an adjunct to appropriate conventional therapy." We also joined Ewan Cameron in recommending that physicians consider administering large amounts of sodium ascorbate by intravenous infusion to patients with advanced cancer. Cameron himself gave intravenous ascorbate, usually 10 grams per day for about 10 days, as well as oral ascorbate continued indefinitely, to each of his patients, and other physicians have reported the successful use of intravenous ascorbate.

Patients started on treatment soon after they have been diagnosed appear to have a better prognosis compared to those who are started several years after they have been diagnosed. This may mean that the treatment they have already had has decreased their ability to respond as well to ortho-molecular treatment. I have examined the relationship between the interval between first symptoms and when patients first consulted me. From this group of 40 female patients, those who started on therapy about the same time as they were started on xenobiotic therapy had a ten month advantage over those who were started after an average of nine months. I have just completed a further evaluation of a larger group, not included in the 134 group. Their follow-up

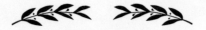

period is less, but comparing the outcome over the three years of follow-up, it is apparent that their outcome will be very similar to the outcome of the previous group.

Skin cancer is becoming more prevalent and has increased the need for better sunscreens. These must protect us against ultraviolet damage. Apparently the ultraviolet light after penetrating the skin increases the formation of free radicals. It therefore makes sense to increase the protection against free radicals by using nature's antioxidants, vitamin C, vitamin E, beta carotene, and selenium. The frequent and recurring reports in the news media about the dangers inherent in excessive exposure to sunlight continually remind and frighten some people about the possibility of getting skin cancer. However, these reports do not discuss the connection between the nutritional health of the population and their susceptibility to cancer of the skin. Since ultraviolet irradiation increases the formation of free radicals, it would not be surprising that increasing the availability of antioxidants would prevent some of the toxic reactions to ultraviolet radiation.

Dr. John Murray, Professor of Dermatology at Duke University, found that vitamin C decreased the intensity of the reaction to ultraviolet light. Subjects were pretreated with a vitamin C solution or with placebo. The protective effect was immediate. The vitamin C was not a sunscreen but it decreased the effect of ultra violet light by its antioxidant properties — that is, it wiped out some of the free radicals that were formed. The fat soluble antioxidant vitamin E should also have protective properties. Dr. Evan Shute reported that vitamin E in ointment or oral form protected against radiation burns. For many years I have been advising friends and family to apply vitamin E cream or to use the contents of the vitamin E capsules to protect themselves against sun burns. Even after they have burned, application of this vitamin has quickly removed the pain and has prevented serious burns. It too acts as an antioxidant.

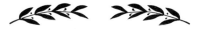

It has been shown that selenium will be such a preventive nutrient. Selenium given to hairless pigmented mice protected them against damage from ultraviolet irradiation. A lotion containing 0.02 percent L-selenomethionine or oral administration of water containing 1.2 p.p.m. both were protective. These dosages did not cause any toxic reactions. This study concluded that "SeMet is effective in protecting against skin cancer induced by UV irradiation, both by retarding the onset and reducing the number of lesions." They were also "effective in reducing the acute damage induced by UV irradiation-inflammation(sunburn), blistering, and pigmentation (tanning)." Selenium is a good antioxidant. It is synergistic with vitamin E, the body's best known fat soluble antioxidant. The daily recommended dose is 200 micrograms. I have given 600 micrograms and more to certain patients for many years and have seen no toxic side effects.

> *I would therefore suggest that the three best known natural antioxidants — ascorbic acid, vitamin E, and selenium — be used to protect people against the toxic effect of excessive ultraviolet irradiation.*

LAW

I would therefore suggest that the three best known natural antioxidants — ascorbic acid, vitamin E, and selenium — be used to protect people against the toxic effect of excessive ultraviolet irradiation. It would be prudent to use optimum amounts of vitamins C and E and selenium and to apply a sunscreen containing all these antioxidants — vitamin C, vitamin E, and selenium. The dose would be 200 micrograms selenium, 800 i.u. of vitamin E, and 3 or more grams per day of ascorbic acid. It should not take too much time to test these antioxidants in controlled studies. But because the danger from ultraviolet induced skin cancer and melanoma is potentially so great, it would appear to me to be prudent to take these simple nutrients as a precaution. They would of course have other advantages as well.

VITAMIN B COMPLEX

Vitamin B complex preparations are available and labeled B-complex 25s, or B-complex 50s or B-complex 75s, or even B-complex 100s. The first one contains 25 mg per tablet of thiamin, riboflavin, nicotinamide, and pyridoxine plus small amounts of the other B vitamins. Similar preparations are called anti-stress vitamins. These are useful preparations made by many drug and vitamin companies. Very few people have any problem with them, though some may be worried about the yellow urine caused by the riboflavin in the preparations. It is a useful marker whether or not the tablet gets absorbed into the body.

These are very useful in ensuring that all the B-vitamins will be provided. They are also very helpful in determining whether vitamins in general are needed. For those who are allergic to yeast the preferred ones are yeast free.

VITAMIN B-1 (*Thiamin*)

The early scientists recognized only two kinds of vitamins, the fat soluble one called vitamin A and the water soluble ones. Thiamin was the first water soluble vitamin to be identified. When more water soluble vitamins were found, they were

Thiamin is essential for the metabolism of carbohydrates. When deficient, the disease beri beri results.

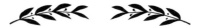

named in order of discovery as B-1, B-2, and later B-3. After their structure was determined they were given their chemical names — thiamin, riboflavin, and nicotinic acid and its amide.

Thiamin is essential for the metabolism of carbohydrates. When deficient, the disease beri beri results. Ironically, thiamin would never have been discovered if it had not been first removed from staple foods. In the Far East white rice became fashionable in this century. White rice is made by polishing off the outer layers of the whole original or brown rice, thereby removing the bran, germ, and adjacent layers. In cereal grains like rice or wheat this is where the major part of the thiamin is located. People living mostly on white rice would suffer a thiamin deficiency or beri beri. The Japanese navy wanted to solve the problem of so many of their sailors having beri beri. This led to the studies that showed that a food factor had been removed, later identified as thiamin. Adding this to the food prevented the disease beri beri. More recently brown rice has been heat treated to drive the thiamin further in so that polishing the rice does not remove as much of the thiamin. Thiamin is one of the vitamins added to white flour in North America. Beri beri is very rare now that thiamin has been restored to processed grains.

There are only a few indications for using large doses of thiamin. Most people will need less than 50 mg daily, the amount that is found in the vitamin B-complex preparations called B Complex-50. The amount available in food due to fortification of white flour will ensure that very few will get beri beri. The exceptions are people who consume large quantities of carbohydrates. They usually are on a diet too rich in refined carbohydrates and fats which provides minimal amounts of all the vitamins and increases the need for thiamin. The best example is alcoholism. Some alcoholics develop a very serious killer disease called Wernicke-Korsakoff syndrome. The recommended treatment for this is to give

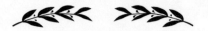

large amounts of thiamin, parenterally at first and later by mouth. Up to 500 mg per day are recommended. I also add vitamin B-3 in large doses to my patients. They respond much better to the combination. This syndrome may be an example of a double dependency, vitamin B-1 and vitamin B-3. After the syndrome has been controlled, smaller amounts of thiamin will keep them well if they stop drinking. I think people who are obese because of their heavy sugar intake would also be helped by extra thiamin. It has been used for some patients with depression.

The therapeutic dose ranges from 50 to 3000 mg daily but the highest doses are very seldom used. Most doses are less than 100 mg daily, except for alcoholics when it will have to go as high as 500 mg. I have given 3 grams per day with no difficulty and no side effects. It may be given by injection as well. As Dr. John Marks notes, "The only reaction found in humans is of the hypersensitivity type. In the vast majority of cases these have occurred after injection of thiamin, and a skin-test dose is advised before undertaking parenteral administration of thiamin in patients with a history of allergic reactions. For parenteral administration the dose that has produced these reactions varies from 5 to 100 mg, although the majority of the reactions occur in the higher part of this range. Since the RDA is 1.4 mg this means the margin of safety is still high. Very rare cases of transient hypersensitivity reactions have also been reported after oral high doses usually in the range of 5 to 10 g (but with one case report at 17 mg). Hence for oral administration the safety factor is at least 100 times the RDA."

A few patients find that on high doses of thiamin there is a thiamin odor on their skin which they find offensive. Others have told me it was also offensive to mosquitoes.

VITAMIN B-2 (*Riboflavin*)

This vitamin is water soluble, easily destroyed by light and

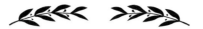

heat. It is also added to white flour. It is yellow with a beautiful fluorescence when exposed to ultra violet light. Very few people are deficient. It has not been studied very intensively. It is helpful in preventing cataracts in elderly patients if the treatment is started very early. This vitamin is effective against carpal tunnel syndrome. There is also a report that phenothiazine tranquilizers will increase the need for riboflavin. The dose ranges from 50 to several hundred mg daily. The majority of people will not need more than 50 mg. There are no side effects with these doses.

VITAMIN B-3 (*Niacin and Niacinamide*)

The third water soluble vitamin to be discovered was the antipellagra vitamin before it was shown to be niacin. I first heard about vitamins in my second year at the university in 1935 in a class called Biochemistry 1. The professor was Roger Manning, a biochemist. He systematically covered all the known vitamins, beginning with vitamin B-1, then vitamin B-2, and later vitamin B-3. But the use of the number B-3 did not stay in the literature very long. It was replaced by nicotinic acid and its amide (also known medically as niacin and niacinamide). The name was changed to remove the similarity to nicotine, a poison. I had a chronic paranoid patient who refused to take nicotinic acid because he thought it was nicotine but who did not object to taking niacin.

The term vitamin B-3 was reintroduced by my friend Mr. Bill W. (Bill Wilson), co-founder of Alcoholics Anonymous. We met in New York in 1960, where my colleague Humphry Osmond and I introduced him to the concept of megavitamin therapy. We described the results we had seen with our schizophrenic patients, some of whom were also alcoholic. We also told him about its many other properties. It was therapeutic for arthritis, for some cases of senility, and it lowered cholesterol levels. Bill was very curious about it and began to take niacin, 3 g daily. Within a few weeks fatigue and

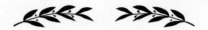

depression which had plagued him for years were gone. He gave it to 30 of his close friends in AA and persuaded them to try it. Within six months he was convinced that it would be very helpful to alcoholics. Of the 30 friends, 10 were free of anxiety, tension, and depression in one month. Another 10 were well in two months. He decided that the chemical or medical terms for this vitamin were not appropriate. He wanted to persuade members of AA, especially the doctors in AA, that this would be a useful addition to treatment and he needed a term that could be more readily popularized. He asked me the names that had been used. I then recalled Professor Manning's lectures and told him it was originally known as vitamin B-3. This was the term Bill wanted. In his first report to physicians in AA he called it "The Vitamin B-3 Therapy." Thousands of copies of this extraordinary pamphlet were distributed. Eventually the name came back and today even the most conservative medical journals are using the term vitamin B-3.

Bill soon became unpopular with the members of the board of AA International. The medical members who had been appointed by Bill felt that he had no business messing about with treatment using vitamins. They also believed vitamin B-3 could not be as therapeutic as Bill had found it to be. For this reason Bill provided information to the medical members of AA outside of the National Board, publishing and distributing three more pamphlets which are still in demand.

Vitamin B-3 exists as the amide in nature, in nicotinamide adenine dinucleotide (NAD). Pure nicotinamide and niacin are synthetics. Niacin was known as a chemical for about 100 years before it was recognized to be vitamin B-3. It is made from nicotine, a poison produced in the tobacco plant to protect itself against its predators, but in the wonderful economy of nature which does not waste any structures, when the nicotine is simplified by cracking open one of the rings it becomes the immensely valuable vitamin B-3.

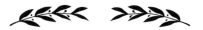

Vitamin B-3 is made in the body from the amino acid tryptophan. On the average 1 mg of vitamin B-3 is made from 60 mg of tryptophan, a 1.5 percent conversion rate. Since it is made in the body it does not meet the strict definition of a vitamin which are defined as substances that cannot be made by the body. It should have been classified with the amino acids but long usage of the term vitamin has given it permanent status as a vitamin. I suspect that one day in the far distant future none of the tryptophan will be converted into vitamin B-3 and it then will truly be a vitamin.

The 1.5 percent conversion rate is a compromise based upon the conversion of tryptophan to N-methyl nicotinamide and its metabolites in human subjects. According to M.K. Horwitt, the amount converted is not inflexible but varies with patients and conditions. For example, women pregnant in their last three months convert tryptophan to niacin metabolites three times as efficiently as in non-pregnant females. Also there is evidence that contraceptive steroids or estrogens stimulate tryptophan oxygenase, the enzyme that converts the tryptophan into niacin.

This observation raises some interesting speculations. Women, on average, live longer then men. It has been shown in men that giving them niacin increases their longevity. Is the increased longevity in women the result of greater conversion of tryptophan into niacin under the stimulus of their increase in estrogen production? Does the same phenomenon explain the lower incidence of coronary disease in women? Elsewhere I have suggested that in schizophrenics there is a decrease in the production of niacin from tryptophan, that this is part of a slow evolutionary change which will one day totally remove this source of niacin, and we will have to depend entirely on external sources. It was observed a long time ago that pregnant women were to a degree less prone to develop schizophrenia, and when it did occur, it often took the form of a post partum psychosis.

The best known vitamin B-3 deficiency disease is pellagra.

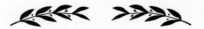

More accurately it is a tryptophan deficiency disease since tryptophan alone can cure the early stages. Pellagra was endemic in the Southern United States until the beginning of the last world war. It can be described by the four D's — dermatitis, diarrhea, dementia, and death. The dementia is a late stage phenomenon. In the early stages it resembles much more the schizophrenias and can only with difficulty be distinguished from it. I consider it one of the schizophrenic syndromes.

Uses

I have been involved in establishing two of the major uses for vitamin B-3, apart from its role in preventing and treating pellagra. These are its action in lowering high cholesterol levels while elevating high density lipoprotein (HDL) cholesterol levels, and its therapeutic role in the schizophrenias and other psychiatric conditions. It has been found helpful for many other diseases or conditions, including learning and behavioral disorders among children, alcoholism and drug addiction, and some of the senile states. It is also a good antidote against d-lysergic acid diethylamide (LSD)intoxication. On the physical side it is useful in improving healing, preventing juvenile diabetes, treating the arthritides, and preventing cardiovascular disease. It has been used to treat kidney disease with success.

Of the two major findings made by my research group in Saskatchewan, the nicotinic acid cholesterol connection is well known, and nicotinic acid is used world wide as an economical, effective, and safe compound for lowering cholesterol and elevating high density lipoprotein cholesterol. However, its therapeutic value in treating schizophrenia has been almost totally ignored by psychiatry in spite of the four double blind controlled experiments we did in the early 1950s and in spite of over 50 papers published in the medical literature by my colleagues and I dealing with various aspects

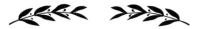

of this treatment. This suggests to me that psychiatry is at least 20 years behind general medicine in adopting new paradigms. Once an idea has been developed it moves pretty readily across the whole field. Thus after the initial strong effort to launch tranquilizers, there is no difficulty moving in as many new ones as the companies are willing to sponsor. I suspect that it will take another 20 years before every schizophrenic is given the benefit of orthomolecular treatment, which includes mainly vitamin B-3 and vitamin B-6. I will therefore include here a much longer discussion of the role this vitamin plays in treating schizophrenic, even chronic, patients who do not respond in a few months but may need several years of treatment in an overall comprehensive program which includes diet, nutrients, and drugs in an optimum combination. In my book *Vitamin B-3 and Schizophrenia: Discovery, Recovery, Controversy*, I have told this story in full.

In 1951 my colleague, Dr. Humphry Osmond, and I developed a unified hypothesis of schizophrenia which united biochemical and psychosocial factors. We suggested that in schizophrenia there was an abnormal production of adrenochrome which then acted on the brain much as does the hallucinogen d-lysergic acid diethylamide (LSD). Adrenochrome is one of the more reactive derivatives of adrenaline. Noradrenochrome is the derivative from noradrenalin. Over the next ten years my research group in Saskatchewan established that adrenochrome is an hallucinogen, that the biochemical conditions necessary for its formation in the body were all present, and that using a compound that blocked its activity on the brain was therapeutic for schizophrenia. That compound was vitamin B-3, either nicotinic acid or nicotinamide. Recently it was shown that adrenochrome is made in the body and there rapidly converted into adrenolutin, a reduced derivative. Both have hallucinogenic properties.

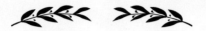

As I developed our research program with Dr. Osmond, we had to meet some opposition from the Canadian professors of psychiatry who did not like our hypothesis and tried to block us from getting research grants. However, with the help of Dr. Nolan D.C. Lewis, then Director of the Psychiatric Institute in New York, we were awarded our first Government of Canada grant in 1952. I was Director of Psychiatric Research for the Province of Saskatchewan. Later we were given a large grant from the Rockefeller Foundation which made it possible to enlarge our research group substantially over the next six years. We then discovered that this vitamin given in gram doses per day lowered cholesterol levels. Since then it has been found that vitamin B-3 also elevates high density lipoprotein cholesterol, thus bringing the ratio of total cholesterol over HDL to below 5. This was a very fortunate finding because it led to the approval by the FDA of this vitamin in mega doses for cholesterol problems and opened up the use of this vitamin in large doses for other conditions as well. This occurred at a time when the FDA was doing its best not to recognize the value of megavitamin therapy.

By 1957 our research group had published a large number of papers dealing with various aspects of psychiatric disease and we were recognized as one of the better research groups in North America. Apart from skepticism of our adrenochrome hypothesis, we did not run into much opposition. This changed, though, after we published our first report that vitamin B-3 was useful for the treatment of acute schizophrenia. Suddenly psychiatry found its basic concepts of schizophrenia challenged as no other finding ever had before. Tranquilizers were being introduced but they were accepted as better sedatives which simply made psychotherapy more effective. This did not run counter to psychodynamic theories which had swept into psychiatry after the last war.

The four double blind controlled studies we did between

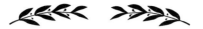

1952 and 1958 showed that adding one vitamin, vitamin B-3, to the current treatment doubled the two year recovery rate from 35 percent to about 75 percent. Since then a large number of studies from our group and from many other practitioners showed that these results were improved by the addition of other nutrients and by more attention to the use of the optimum diets for these patients. Still, our earlier studies were not promising for the chronic patients. Vitamin B-3 therapy, as the single vitamin, did not appear to help chronic patients. Later I found that if the treatment was combined with other treatment and maintained for several years the results were more promising.

Recently I examined the outcome of treatment of 27 chronic patients who remained under my care for ten years and more. They were ill on the average seven years before they came under my treatment program. This is only a relatively small portion of the large number of chronic patients I am treating. The average age of this group was 40 years when they started the program, they had failed to respond to all previous treatments, and they were still following the program. This consisted of a good diet, the correct vitamin and mineral supplements, and medication such as tranquilizers and antidepressants as required. My survey showed that today 11 are working, two are married and looking after their families, two are single mothers caring for their children with no difficulty, three are managing their own business. One patient received his B.Sc. from the local university, one was awarded her M.A., another got a certificate from the community college. From this total group today 18 are well, three are much improved, five are improved. None are worse.

Using the best xenobiotic therapy, it is clear that from a similar group of chronic patients one would expect almost no cases of recovery, while at best a few might have reached an improved state. As reported in *The British Journal of Psychiatry*, E.C. Johnston and his colleagues studied 532 schizophrenic patients treated over a 10 year period beginning in 1975 for

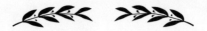

their recovery rates. It was found that only two patients were now in the best occupational levels (this means that they were well) and 25 were found in the next best occupational level. That is, only five percent of this large group had shown any significant recovery. They found that close contact between patients and their treating doctors did not improve the results any — closer supervision was not helpful. They even questioned whether there was any benefit to closer monitoring of these patients. This large group must have included a large number of acute and chronic patients. Only their most chronic patients would be comparable to the 26 described in my report.

In the 1970s I treated the sick daughter of a prominent New York resident who had been diagnosed as having schizophrenia. She became ill after graduating from a women's college. She began to experience hallucinations and became obsessive. She was admitted to hospital, treated with electro shock therapy (ECT), and tranquilizers. At the end, after having spent $250,000 vintage 1975 dollars, she was catatonic. Over the next five years she was treated in seven hospitals by a number of top specialists. The parents consulted me and I advised them to start her on our vitamin B-3 program. In discussing what I thought was the most correct diagnosis for this condition, I pointed out that it closely resembled the psychosis of pellagra and that in my opinion was a variant of it — it was a vitamin B-3 dependency. This appealed to the parents' good sense and they began to look upon it as a form of pellagra. After my discussion with the family, they discovered that just before she graduated she had gone onto a crash diet supported by medically prescribed amphetamines, losing 12 pounds weekly. After she was started on the orthomolecular program I recommended to them, she began to recover and remains well.

Our finding that this vitamin helped schizophrenics but only when used in large doses also challenged the nutritional establishment which was still preoccupied with the idea that

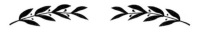

the average balanced diet was so good it did not need to be supplemented, and secondly that taking any quantity of vitamin above these small doses would be ineffective since the extra amounts would be excreted in the urine. Their view of vitamins was very primitive. Thus our report stirred up a massive amount of criticism based almost entirely upon theoretical ideas and not upon clinical research.

We were surprised by the extent of the opposition but accepted it as the inevitable result of promoting new ideas in medicine. New ideas historically have had to run the gauntlet of opposition for up to 40 years before they are incorporated into the body of medicine. I was surprised by the intensity of the opposition but I was astounded by the vigor and hostility of the attack upon us personally. This was a major factor in my decision to leave my two jobs, as Research Director and as Associate Professor of Psychiatry, University of Saskatchewan. The debate broke several relationships between myself and colleagues with whom I had been very friendly. But there were only two attempts by official medical bodies to prevent us from doing our work.

Soon after I opened my practice of psychiatry in Saskatoon, I helped organize the Saskatchewan Schizophrenia Association and became its first president. We had no money and started with a bank loan which I co-signed. To raise money I sent a form letter to every doctor in Saskatchewan telling them about the association and requesting financial support. A few months later I received a letter from the College of Physicians and Surgeons of Saskatchewan. This was the body which controlled licensure of all physicians in Saskatchewan. Apparently a psychiatrist had complained to them that I has engaging in public advertising by sending out that appeal letter. Before I went to the hearing I thought I was being jumped upon because I was promoting treatment views that other psychiatrists found unacceptable. I went to the meeting prepared to defend the work that I was doing. Later I discovered the real reason. A

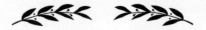

member of the College with whom I was friendly told me later that if I had not signed that letter they would not have called me. Advertising was considered by the college a greater sin than raping one's patient. They took a very narrow view of this. I was given a mild reprimand. But behind that attempt at censure was the psychiatric dislike of our view that vitamins could be helpful in treating schizophrenia and perhaps antagonism toward the Saskatchewan Schizophrenia Association which was promoting the view that vitamins were helpful.

The American Psychiatric Association attempted to suppress our work several years later. I had published a paper in 1967 describing the results of treatment on five California patients. The patients had failed to respond to the best treatment they could get in California, including psychoanalysis, family therapy, medication, and so on. One of them came to me for treatment and the rest were treated in California by orthomolecular physicians. They all recovered. One of this group is now a research psychiatrist. Following this publication a couple of California psychiatrists complained to the American Psychiatric Association that we were promulgating treatments not acceptable to the profession. I received a letter from the APA advising me that this kind of behavior was unacceptable. I was then a Fellow of this association. They had no power or any authority over me, nor could they have in any way injured me or the practice. However, I was irritated by this attempt to suppress our work. I discovered that APA had not followed its own constitution and bylaws in sending me this mild censure. The matter should have come before the Committee on Ethics or even better before its Scientific Affairs Committee. These committees had not been consulted. I wrote back demanding that they follow proper procedure and that they must let me know the nature of the charges against me (and Dr. Osmond) as well as the name of the persons who had laid the complaint. Eventually they told me it was about that article but they would not divulge who had complained. They agreed to meet with Dr. Osmond and

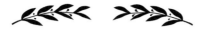

I early in the 1970s in Washington to answer the charges. I was astonished at the ineptitude of the committee who apparently had not made any attempt to read our papers. They knew nothing about our work. At the end of a rather heated morning discussion they announced they would let us have their decision in a few days. I had protested vigorously their right to even investigate us, pointing out that we were engaged in a scientific debate, and we had not been unethical in promulgating views for which we had ample evidence.

We have still not heard from the APA. They concluded they had no case but were too cowardly to let us know this, or else they were fearful that we would announce that we had been investigated by them and that they had not found us to be unethical. The main result was that I then resigned from the APA because I did not relish the idea that my annual fee as a Fellow would be used against me.

The onus is now on orthodox psychiatry to demonstrate by research of their own that there is a major fault in our conclusions. It is not good enough to assume that this is all due to a series of unproved assumptions such as a placebo effect, faith, or even some monstrous conspiracy to show something works when in fact it does not. Or will the profession adopt the stance of a California psychiatrist who recently testified for 15 minutes before a judge that one of the patients was psychotic since she believed that vitamins had been helpful to her? World psychiatry experienced similar types of reasoning and conclusions from Russian psychiatrists who labeled dissidents psychotic simply because they were dissidents.

> *Our major problem today is the slow pace of recognition of new therapeutic ideas in medicine and especially in psychiatry. Until now it has taken anywhere from 40 to 60 years for new treatments to be generally accepted. This is very costly.*
>
> LAW

Our major problem today is the slow pace of recognition of new therapeutic ideas in medicine and especially in

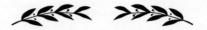

psychiatry. Until now it has taken anywhere from 40 to 60 years for new treatments to be generally accepted. This is very costly. Thus the British Navy began to issue limes to their sailors 40 years *after* Dr. James Lind proved that oranges and lemons cured and prevented scurvy. During those 40 years the Navy lost 100,000 seamen from scurvy. How many schizophrenics today are being condemned to permanent and debilitating disease for the rest of their lives because of this slow pace in accepting new treatments. We must develop a mechanism by which new discoveries are promptly used in all of medicine. This should not be beyond the wit of humanity. It could be done very economically and with scientific precision if only there was the will to do so.

Optimum Dose

The optimum dose range for vitamin B-3 is not as wide as it is for ascorbic acid, but it is wide enough to require different recommendations for different classes of diseases. As is always the case with nutrients, individuals must determine their own optimum. With nicotinic acid, this is done by increasing the doses until the flush (vasodilatation) is gone or is so slight it is not a problem. One can start with as low a dose as 100 mg taken three times each day after meals and gradually increase it. I usually start with 500 mg each dose and often will start with 1 gram per dose especially for cases of arthritis, for schizophrenics, for alcoholics, and for a few elderly patients. However, with elderly patients it is better to start small and work it up slowly.

No person should be given nicotinic acid without explaining to them that they will have a flush which will vary in intensity from none to very severe. If this is explained carefully and if they are told that in time the flush will not be a problem, they will not mind. The flush may remain too intense for a few patients and the nicotinic acid may have to be replaced by a slow release preparation or by some of the esters, for example, inositol niacinate. The latter is a very

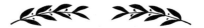

good preparation with very little flush and most find it very acceptable even when they were not able to accept the nicotinic acid itself. It is rather expensive but with quantity production the price might come down.

The flush starts in the forehead with a warning tingle. Then it intensifies. The rate of the development of the flush depends upon so many factors it is impossible to predict what course it will follow. The following factors decrease the intensity of the flush: a cold meal, taking it after a meal, taking aspirin before, using an antihistamine in advance. The following factors make the flush more intense: a hot meal, a hot drink, an empty stomach, chewing the tablets, and the rate at which the tablets break down in liquid. From the forehead and face the flush travels down the rest of the body, usually stopping somewhere in the chest but may extend to the toes. With continued use the flush gradually recedes and eventually may be only a tingling sensation in the forehead. If the person stops taking the vitamin for a day or more the sequence of flushing will be re-experienced. Some people never do flush and a few only begin to flush after several years of taking the vitamin. With nicotinamide there should be no flushing, but I have found that about two percent will flush. This may be due to rapid conversion of the nicotinamide to nicotinic acid in the body.

When the dose is too high for both forms of the vitamin, the patients will suffer from nausea at first, and if the dose is not reduced, from vomiting. These side effects may be used to determine what is the optimum dose. When they do occur, the dose is reduced until it is just below the nausea level. With children the first indication may be loss of appetite. If this does occur, the vitamin must be stopped for a few days and then may resumed at a lower level. Very few can take more than 6 grams per day of the nicotinamide. With nicotinic acid it is possible to go much higher. Many schizophrenics have taken up to 30 grams per day with no difficulty. The dose will alter over time and if on a dose

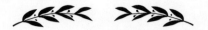

where there were no problems, they may develop in time. Usually this indicates that the patient is getting better and does not need as much.

For people who are well or nearly well and have no obvious disease, who are interested in maintaining their good health or in improving it, who may be under increased stress, the optimum dose of nicotinic acid varies between 1 and 3 grams daily. The same doses apply to nicotinamide. For everyone under physiological stress, such as pregnancy and lactation, suffering from acute illness, such as the common cold or flu or other diseases that do not threaten immediate death, the dose range is 1 gram to 10 grams daily for nicotinic acid, 1.5 g to 6 grams for nicotinamide. All the psychiatric syndromes are included in this group, including the schizophrenias and the senile states. It also includes the very large group of people with high blood cholesterol levels or low HDL when it is desired to restore these blood values to normal.

The side-effects of taking vitamin B-3 in niacin or nicotinic form have been described by Dr. John Marks as follows: "A tingling or flushing sensation in the skin after relatively large doses (in excess of 75 mg) of nicotinic acid is a rather common phenomenon. It is the result of dilatation of the blood vessels that is one of the natural actions of nicotinic acid and one for which it is used therapeutically. Whether this should therefore be regarded as a true adverse reaction is a moot point. The reaction clears regularly after about 20 minutes and is not harmful to the individual. It is very rare for this reaction to occur at less than three times the RDA, even in very sensitive individuals. In most people much larger quantities are required. The related substance nicotinamide only very rarely produces this reaction and in consequence this is the form generally used for vitamin supplementation.

"Doses of 200 mg to 10 g daily of the acid have been used therapeutically to lower blood cholesterol levels under medical control for periods of up to 10 years or more and though

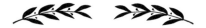

some reactions have occurred at these very high dosages, they have rapidly responded to cessation of therapy, and have often cleared even when therapy has been continued.

"In isolated cases, transient liver disorders, rashes, dry skin and excessive pigmentation have been seen. The tolerance to glucose has been reduced in diabetics and patients with peptic ulcers have experienced increased pain. No serious reaction have been reported however even in these high doses. The available evidence suggests that 100 times the RDA is safe (about 100 mg)."

Dr. Marks is cautious about recommending that doses over 100 mg are safe. In my opinion, based upon 40 years of experience with this vitamin, the dose ranges I have recommended are safe. However, with the higher doses medical supervision is necessary. As well, you should avoid using slow release preparations which may cause hepatitis or jaundice and even more serious problems. Jaundice is very rare. Fewer that 10 cases have been reported in the medical literature, and I have seen none in 10 years. When jaundice does occur, it is usually an obstructive type and clears when the vitamin is discontinued. I have been able to get schizophrenic patients back on nicotinic acid after the jaundice cleared and it did not recur. Since jaundice in people who have not been taking nicotinic acid is fairly common, it is possible there is a random association. The liver function tests may indicate there is a problem when in fact there is not. Nicotinic acid should be stopped for five days before the liver function tests are given. There have been three cases of severe liver damage attributed to slow release preparations, though, and of these three one patient died, another needed a liver transplant. One patient who had no problem with nicotinic acid for lowering cholesterol switched to the slow release preparations and became ill. When he resumed the original nicotinic acid, he was well again with no further evidence of liver dysfunction. I have not seen any cases reported anywhere else.

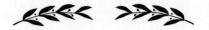

VITAMIN B-6 (*Pyridoxine*)

Vitamin B-6 is the second major vitamin of the water soluble B series which has been studied by orthomolecular physicians. A major impetus was given to this study by Dr. C.C. Pfeiffer when he discovered that in the absence of enough pyridoxine and zinc, there was in many patients an increase in the excretion of a substance in the urine called kryptopyrrole (KP). This compound was first found in the urine of schizophrenic patients by our research group. In looking for a unique compound which might be present in the urine of schizophrenics, we tested the urine of a non schizophrenic alcoholic who was given LSD. After he took the LSD, he began to excrete large amounts of a substance that turned pink on a paper chromatogram when it was developed with the correct chemicals. Later we found that this compound, which we called the mauve factor, was present in the majority of early schizophrenic patients, and that when they become well, it was no longer present. Dr. Pfeiffer found that when it was present there was also a double deficiency of zinc and pyridoxine. When these two nutrients were given in adequate doses, the kryptopyrrole disappeared.

Uses

There are several good reasons for using pyridoxine therapeutically, both for psychiatric patients and for patients with physical disease.

Schizophrenics, many children with learning and behavioral disorders, and children with infantile autism often excrete large amounts of KP. The urine test for KP is relatively simple and any modern laboratory can learn to do it with little difficulty. Dr. Bernard Rimland, who was a co-worker in the first double blind prospective controlled experiment which showed that pyridoxine was therapeutic for these children, has stated that "there are now 17 published studies — all positive — showing that high dosages of

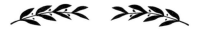

vitamin B-6 and magnesium are a safe and often helpful treatment for autism. Thousands of parents are using B-6 and magnesium to help their children. Almost 50 percent show worthwhile improvement and the vitamins are immeasurably safer than any drug."

Dr. John Marion Ellis and Dr. Karl Folkers concluded that vitamin B-6, 50-200 mg taken daily for 12 weeks, cured the less affected hand in patients suffering from carpal tunnel syndrome who were selected for surgery on the more crippled hand. The vitamin B-6 treatment halted atrophy of the thenar muscle. They suggested it is a co-factor for normal cortisone activity in tendons and synovium. They also reported one case where riboflavin alone was very effective in treating carpal tunnel syndrome, but when both vitamin B-2 and B-6 were given together, the results were even better. They concluded that this syndrome was the result of a double vitamin deficiency.

The double deficiency of vitamin B-6 and zinc produces symptoms in the skin, including stretch marks on the body and white spots in the finger nails. These are not calcium spots. When the two nutrients are provided, they clear. Premenstrual syndrome also responds well to these two nutrients.

Pyridoxine is receiving increasing attention as a nutrient involved in protection against arteriosclerosis, heart disease, and strokes. It is one of the nutrients essential in the conversion of homocysteine to the non-toxic cystathionine. I have discussed this under folic acid, another of these essential nutrients. Interest in the relation between pyridoxine and the development of atherosclerosis was aroused by the pioneer work of a physician practicing in Johannesburg, South Africa. Dr. Moses M. Suzman, an internist, had theorized that atherosclerosis was a vitamin deficiency disease. He suspected multiple vitamin and mineral deficiencies, primarily vitamin B-6. In his study, he administered to patients pyridoxine 200 mg, folic acid 5 mg, and vitamin E 100 to 600 i.u., all daily. He also used other nutrients in smaller amounts.

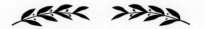

Of 62 typical heart patients followed for an average of 52 months, there were four reinfarcts (two were fatal). Dr. J.M. Ellis, who had been using pyridoxine for a long time to treat carpal tunnel syndrome with great success, observed that few of his patients on this vitamin had heart attacks. Dr. Suzman was not able to publish his main body of data in medical journals, however, because they found his ideas too novel. I am familiar with these difficulties since we ran into the same problem publishing our vitamin B-3 schizophrenia data over the past 20 years. It is generally not known to the public that the peer review system of vetting papers to be published in medical journals effectively suppresses any idea the "peers" do not like. In fact, they are not even "peers" since they are not informed about the treatment, nor have they been taught anything about it as medical students.

Dose

For people who are well or nearly well and who wish to ensure they will have enough, I recommend 50 to 100 mg daily. For specific indications of deficiency or disease, I recommend between 100 and 500 mg daily. Larger doses have been used but they are seldom needed. In children it may be necessary to also use magnesium to prevent the pyridoxine from activating hyperactive behavior in the child. This observation, first reported by Adelle Davis in one of her books, has been confirmed by many.

Side Effects

There are very few. The ones that do occur are minor and transient. Much has been made of the few patients collected from several medical schools who took between 2000 and 6000 mg per day. These patients developed a peripheral neuropathy which cleared after a year. But based on this report the idea became current that vitamin B-6 was toxic. Dr. John Marks has proven otherwise: "It has been claimed

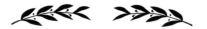

that high doses of pyridoxine can lead to liver damage, interference with the normal functions of riboflavin and a dependency state. With the possible exception of the dependency states these suggestions are not substantiated by scientific data. The dependency states were very transient."

PANTOTHENIC ACID, FOLIC ACID, VITAMIN B-12 (*Cobalamin*)

These three vitamins have not been examined as thoroughly by orthomolecular physicians. It is likely that when a proper search is made, there will be patients who are found to be dependent upon them, and who if identified, could be treated successfully.

Pantothenic acid, once known as vitamin B-5, is very safe with no known side effects. Up to 10 to 12 g per day have been given with only occasional diarrhea and water retention. In animals it has been shown to extend life. It has been used to help control food allergies and as a mild anti-anxiety or anti-tension substance. It deserves to be studied in more detail. The optimum doses have not been determined.

Folic acid is another safe water soluble vitamin. It has been used in doses up to 15 mg daily. There has been a report that this dose caused gastrointestinal disturbances but in another study with the same dose this was not seen. Most patients do not need more than 5 mg. Recently it has been proven that women will give birth to babies with spina bifida and similar neural tube defects (NTD) much less frequently if they take supplemental folic acid, 1 mg. I generally recommend 5 mg daily. Dr. Smithells in 1981 showed that giving pregnant women extra folic acid decreased the incidence of NTDs. Before that he had measured the red cell folate and white cell vitamin C levels of mothers who had babies with NTDs and found they were lower in both. It was thus known since 1981 that a multivitamin preparation containing folic

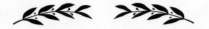

acid would decrease the birth of these damaged babies.

The immediate reaction to the original findings was one of strong disbelief and hostility; the establishment refused to advise women to take folic acid until the requisite number of double blind experiments were done. Almost a decade later the *Journal of the American Medical Association* published a report proving that folic acid provided protection for most causes of the defect. Even in women with a family history of NTD where the frequency of babies with the defects was more than five times greater than normal — 18 per 1000 against 3.5 per 1000 — this treatment was effective. How many babies could have been saved by such a simple solution? Even if the original findings had been wrong, what harm would it have done to have advised them immediately about this very important finding? I was astonished in 1981 at the vehemence of the reaction by physicians and nutritionists.

I am still astonished, especially so when recent studies show that folic acid can decrease NTDs by 75 percent. If all the other vitamins were used as well, I am certain that figure would be closer to 100 percent. I cannot recall in the past 40 years a single female patient of mine on vitamins giving birth to any child with a congenital defect. I have been able to advise them all that they not only would not harm their developing baby by taking vitamins, but that their chances of giving birth to a defective child would be greatly diminished. I was frequently asked this by my patients who had been told by their doctors that they must stop all their vitamins while pregnant. They looked upon vitamins as toxic drugs. I am still asked the same question for the same reason today. However, governments can learn and do respond. It is now official that pregnant women should take extra folic acid in order to prevent spina bifida and other birth defects. The U.S. Public Health Service has issued the following advisory: "In order to reduce the frequency of NTDs (neural-tube defects) and their resulting disability, the United States Public Health Service recommends that: All women of childbearing age

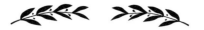

capable of becoming pregnant should consume 0.4 mg of folic acid per day for the purpose of reducing their risk of having a pregnancy affected with spina bifida or other NTDs." This amount will not be provided by most diets and requires supplementation. Apparently the U.S. Public Health Service is considering fortifying bread with folic acid. Folic acid is destroyed by heat but some will survive.

Health and Welfare Canada is more cautious. It recommends that "as early as possible when planning a pregnancy women should consult their physician about folic acid supplements. Women with a previous NTD affected pregnancy are at higher risk of having another affected pregnancy. These women should consult their physician about folic acid supplements. All women of child-bearing potential should follow *Canada's Food Guide to Healthy Eating* and take care to choose more foods higher in folate. For protection against occurrence, 0.4 mg folic acid, alone is likely to be beneficial and not toxic." This advice is problematic because many women do not realize they are pregnant until it is too late for the folic acid to have done any good. It is obvious that Health and Welfare Canada is unaware how little doctors know about vitamins. Consulting them will probably elicit the advice that no vitamins should be taken during pregnancy. Health and Welfare also has less faith in the people of Canada than has the U.S. Public Health Service in the intelligence of the U.S. public.

Folic acid is also one of the nutrients involved in the prevention of arteriosclerosis. Arteriosclerosis is such a complicated phenomenon it is not surprising a large number of factors are involved, including ascorbic acid, nicotinic acid, pyridoxine, and choline. J. Challem in his "The Nutrition Reporter" reviewed the recent literature which suggests that the common factor is homocysteine, which in the body is quickly changed to cystathionine. High levels of homocysteine are now recognized as a risk factor in heart disease. Dr. M. Stampfer analyzed blood from 14,916 male physicians, all of

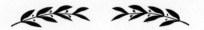

whom had not had a heart attack. Five years later 271 had suffered heart attacks. Of these 31 had extremely high blood levels of homocysteine. Several other studies have found the same relationship. A study at Oregon Health Sciences Center showed that 40 percent of patients who had a stroke had high homocysteine levels. In a normal population it is elevated in five percent. There was an inverse correlation between homocysteine and intake of vitamins. Folic acid is one of the vitamins needed for the rapid conversion of homocysteine to the non-toxic cystathionine. A recent study showed that half of the American population does not get enough folic acid. One to 5 mg of folic acid should be taken daily. This is enough to decrease elevated homocysteine levels in blood.

Folic acid has been found to decrease the odds of getting lung cancer. It has also been shown to reverse changes found in the cervix as measured by the Pap smear; patients with low folate levels are more likely to develop cervical dysplasia. I use it for these reasons. Another indication I have found is in elderly patients who develop a hand tremor which makes it difficult for them to write. Giving them folic acid 5 to 10 mg daily will often remove this problem in a week or so. There is a remote danger that giving folic acid will mask a vitamin B-12 deficiency, pernicious anemia, but a vitamin B-12 blood level will show whether this is a problem. Recently, I have seen what folic acid can do for an elderly male who had been a little more unsteady and who had to be more careful in walking because of this. He had also infrequent episodes of tachycardia which responded in a few minutes to changes in body position, and at other times his pulse rate was too slow and too unresponsive to demand by exercise. He had been on niacin for many years. The addition of 15 mg of folic acid, twice daily, changed this dramatically. The unsteadiness was gone within one hour, and the tachycardia no longer occurred. The low pulse rate has been slowly improving and is no longer a problem on most days.

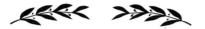

The deficiency of folic acid is also clearly related to psychopathology. Folic acid deficiency is high in patients with depression, senility, and schizophrenia and in epileptic patients on dilantin. Medical patients with folic acid deficiency suffer more from psychiatric symptoms. The addition of folic acid to the diet of these patients produces substantial improvement.

Dr. Paul Godfrey, Institute of Psychiatry, London, has reported that folic acid speeded recovery from depression. One third of their depressed patients were folate deficient. The overall outcome of folic acid therapy was impressive. Every one improved to some extent. The best results were obtained at three to six months. Patients given 10 mg daily responded in two to three months but gastrointestinal and neurological symptoms were improved in five months on 10 mg weekly. It is clear that orthomolecular therapists will have to give much more attention to this important vitamin.

Vitamin B-12 (cobalamin) is absorbed from the intestine, except in patients with pernicious anemia who cannot do so. It is usually given by injection, but recent evidence shows that giving tablets or sublingual lozenges will be as effective. Up to 100 mg per day have been given with no side effects. Vitamin B-12 has been used in megadoses by many physicians for many years for their patients with chronic fatigue, even though their blood levels are normal. There is no doubt that these patients have benefited. Injecting 1000 ug per day provides 1000 times the recommended daily dose.

Other B vitamins include Biotin, Choline, Inositol, Amygdalin (Vitamin B-17), Para-aminobenzoic Acid (PABA), and Pangamic Acid (Vitamin B-15). Their presence in common foods is described later in this book in the chapter on "The Nutrient Content of Foods."

VITAMIN E
(THE TOCOPHEROLS)

Vitamin E was discovered in 1922 (a deficiency caused fetal death and resorption in rats), and pure vitamin E was first isolated from wheat germ oil in 1936. It has only recently become popular. For long it was laughed at as a vitamin in search of a disease. Now we know it prevents us from having many diseases. Vitamin E deficiency, in a classical sense, is found mainly in premature infants, where it causes increased hemolysis of red blood cells and a decreased red blood half life. In adults, it regulates platelet aggregability, prevents peripheral vascular disease, and modulates the immune system.

There are eight naturally occurring forms of vitamin E, of which alpha tocopherol is one of the most active and the one generally used. Vitamin E is present in two forms, the d- form which is the only one with biological activity, and the l- form which has little activity. The synthetic preparation contains equal parts of the d- and l- form and is labeled as dl-alpha tocopherol. It is too expensive to remove the l-form from the synthetic mixture. The d-form is much more expensive because it is extracted from natural sources. There is still some debate about the relative merits of the d- versus the dl-form, but I am convinced that the d-form is more active. I have seen it help people when the same dose of the dl-form

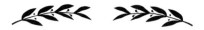

did not. One mg of dl-alpha-tocopherol is designated as 1 International Unit (i.u.); d-alpha-tocopherol is more active and one mg is equivalent to 1.49 i.u.

Vitamin E is a fat soluble vitamin. It is absorbed into the walls of the intestine, there combined with other fats into chylomicrons and distributed throughout the body. It is almost all carried in the low density and high density lipoproteins. Its major role is its scavenger function of free radicals. Free radicals are highly reactive fractions of molecules which, if allowed to remain, will damage cell membranes and amino acids rich in sulfur. Vitamin E is nature's best antioxidant for protecting cell surfaces. One vitamin E molecule will be used over and over and can protect against 1000 free radical molecules.

> *Vitamin E is nature's best antioxidant for protecting cell surfaces. One vitamin E molecule will be used over and over and can protect against 1000 free radical molecules.* **LAW**

The history of vitamin E, its early massive rejection for about 40 years and its increasing acceptance today, contains many lessons for physicians and for medical schools. In the 1940s, two Canadian doctors, the brothers Wilfred and Evan Shute, pioneered research in the therapeutic use of vitamin E, but found their work rejected in large by the medical community chiefly because physicians at that time knew hardly anything about vitamins. Dr. Wilfred and Evan Shute were deprived of any recognition which was deservedly theirs. At the end of their lives they had some satisfaction from the recognition they received from orthomolecular physicians. They were the first doctors who had to face the unreasonable and unrelenting opposition of the medical establishment for their espousal of megadoses of a vitamin. This opposition was totally unscientific. Unless we learn from history we are condemned to repeat this mistake.

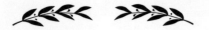

Uses

Vitamin B-3 was the first vitamin used in megadoses in the 1930s, with doses of 600 mg given daily to prevent the symptoms of chronic pellagra from recurring, followed by Dr. William Kaufman's work showing that this vitamin was therapeutic for the arthritides in doses of 3 to 6 grams a daily. Vitamin E was the second vitamin used in these large doses. The Shute brothers in Ontario used 800 i.u. and more to treat large numbers of patients with circulatory problems and heart disease and to accelerate healing after burns. They were subjected to powerful opposition from the medical establishment, especially in Ontario. Medical journals would not publish their papers, so they published in their own journal called *The Summary*. The December 1973 issue contained a report by Evan Shute, as well as letters, abstracts, and striking color photographs of the response of wounds caused by freezing, by diabetes, and by burns to the administration of vitamin E. Dr. Shute, in this issue, described six therapeutic properties of vitamin E. (1) It is both an antioxidant and improves the ability of tissue to use oxygen. (2) It prevents the formation of emboli from clots and extension of the clot. (3) It is a vasodilator for the capillaries. (4) It improves damaged capillary fragility. (5) It resolves some scars. (6) It may improve muscle power in athletes and in animals. Not surprisingly, it has been found to be therapeutic for managing thrombosis, gangrene, indolent ulcers, thromboangiitis obliterans, thermal burns, radiation burns, cardiac disease, congenital heart disease, acute and chronic rheumatic fever, hypertensive heart disease, coronary heart disease. Dr. Shute refers to 57 published reports on the efficacy of vitamin E.

More recently, Vitamin E has been shown to be valuable in the treatment of cardiovascular disease; premenstrual syndrome; and tissue ischemia (common in myocardial infarction, stroke and renal failure). Vitamin E reduces ischemia and will be very important in dealing with these conditions. It has also been shown to be valuable in the prevention of

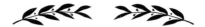

cancer (studies show an inverse relationship between vitamin E status and the development or risk of dying from cancer.); in protection against environmental pollutants (it suppressed increased lipid peroxidation in cigarette smokers); and in enhancing immune functions. It is clear that vitamin E will play an ever increasing role in the prevention and treatment of disease. It is no longer a vitamin in search of a disease. It is now recognized as an antioxidant vitamin intimately involved in the biochemistry and physiology of the body and with a host of diseases. The lay vitamin literature is now well acquainted with vitamin E and its usefulness. In 1972 Dr. E. Di Cyan, a friend of mine, wrote his excellent book *Vitamin E and Aging*, which today is still very up-to-date. He foreshadowed the many current interests of the medical profession which at the time were totally ignored or laughed at.

In November 1992, *New York Newsday* carried a report that vitamin E decreases the risk of heart disease between one-third and one-half. Two studies were conducted at the Harvard School of Public Health. In one study Dr. M. Stampfer and colleagues found that during an eight year follow up, women who had taken at least 100 i.u. of vitamin E daily for two years had a 46 percent lower risk of having a heart attack. This was based on a population study involving 87,245 women. The second study on men by Dr. E. Rimm and colleagues, based upon 51,529 subjects, showed a 37 percent lower risk. Both research teams found that there was not enough vitamin E in food to reach these daily levels. Dr. Stampfer was so convinced by the data that he is himself taking the vitamin.

These findings are not surprising to anyone familiar with the research conducted by Dr. Wilfred Shute and Dr. Evan Shute on over 30,000 patients. However, neither Stampfer nor Rimm and their colleagues in their two papers make any reference to the pioneering work done much earlier by the Shute brothers. Their work was a model of good clinical research but the idea was so novel it was totally ignored and

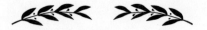

attacked. They were considered quacks since everyone knew that vitamin E had no value for anything. The medical profession, instead of investigating these claims carefully, persisted in downgrading the work.

Today, approximately 40 percent of all deaths in North America are caused by heart disease. Each day 2,000 people die from heart disease. Let us assume that the reduction in risk is exaggerated, and that in reality there is only a 10 percent reduction with therapeutic doses of vitamin E. This means that each day about 200 fewer people would die. It is difficult to calculate overall how many would have been saved if the Harvard group has taken their responsibility seriously and examined the vitamin E claims in 1950 instead of waiting until 1992. This is the real cost of medical cynicism. Had they been merely skeptical, they could have done the studies to satisfy their own curiosity, but they were so convinced the Shutes' findings were meaningless they went out of their way to destroy them. They succeeded. The medical establishment consoles itself by claiming that the onus for proving new findings is on the original investigator. This is merely an excuse for doing nothing. The price is enormous. How much longer will society permit doctors the luxury of doing nothing, especially when the suggested treatments are safe, economical, and, in the opinion of doctors who follow the treatments, so effective.

Two recent reports show that vitamin E also helps heart patients get well after by-pass surgery and angioplasties. Dr. D.S. Sgoutas at Emory University found that 35.5 percent of angioplasty patients taking vitamin E suffered from restenosis, while 47.5 percent of the control placebo group did. Dr. T. Yau at The University of Toronto reported that presurgical supplementation of vitamin E helped the heart pump during the high-risk five-hour postoperative period. Controls did not do as well.

Vitamin E may be working its way into psychiatry following reports that it had a slight effect in decreasing the

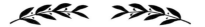

symptoms of tardive dyskinesia in patients. This aroused some to consider its role there as an antioxidant and its possible effect in decreasing the oxidation of catechol amines to their oxidized derivatives. These are compounds like adrenochrome. It is an interesting hypothesis and corroborates our views published in the mid 1950s.

Finally, *The American Journal of Epidemiology* recently reported that people who took vitamin E regularly for at least six months had half the expected risk of oral cancer. This is based upon 1100 patients with oral cancer and 1300 normal controls. The amount of vitamin in multivitamins was not enough; they had to take pure vitamin E supplements, at least 100 i.u. per day. Several other similar studies are underway.

Dose

Dr. W. Shute and E. Shute recommended doses from 400 i.u. to 8000 i.u. daily. The usual dose range was 800 to 1600 i.u. but they report that they had given 8000 i.u. (about 8 grams) without seeing any toxicity. I usually use between 400 and 1200 i.u. daily, but for Crohns disease have been giving 4000 i.u. I have not yet seen any side effects from vitamin E administration. Dr. Marks reports that adults can safely be given 100 to 800 i.u. but excludes adults with alteration of vitamin K status or metabolism. Ingestion of 1,200 i.u. has increased the coagulation defect produced by vitamin K deficiency or by warfarin treatment. Dr. Shute advises starting with small doses for patients who have rheumatic heart disease. He starts with 90 i.u. and very slowly works up the dose. The reason for this is that if too much is given at the beginning the increased strength of the heart beat may create some difficulty. The same applies to heart failure from hypertension. The initial dose should be small and gradually increased. If this is done, the final dose can safely reach 800 to 1200 i.u.

VITAMIN A (CAROTENES)

V itamin A is another fat soluable vitamin which is stored
in the body. It is found in two forms, as retinol in animal foods and as carotene in plant foods primarily.

Over 400 carotenoids are known in nature. They are the
colored pigments widely found in plants. Beta carotene is
the most abundant and best known. One molecule can be
converted into vitamin A. Only about 10 to 50 percent of the
beta carotene consumed is absorbed. The amount changed
to vitamin A depends upon the vitamin state of the body. If
the body has enough vitamin A, no more beta carotene is
converted into the vitamin. It is one of the three major
antioxidants and is therefore receiving more and more attention in the treatment of cancer. It is non toxic. Even with
very high doses the only side effect has been the deposition
of the pigment into the skin and the subjects become a bit
carrot like in color. The extra amounts over normal needs
cannot be converted into vitamin A.

Beta carotene inhibits the formation of tumors in animals, and in human subjects the more beta carotene there
is in their body the less risk there is of getting cancer. By 1989
six studies on cancer of the esophagus showed there was a
positive relationship, eight studies on stomach cancer were
positive, and five studies out of 10 on colon cancer showed
the same connection. There is a similar relationship to heart

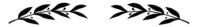

disease. A School of Public Health study showed that women who consumed more than 15-20 mg (25,000 i.u.) daily had a 40 percent less chance of having a heart attack. Cataracts also are found more frequently in people with lower beta carotene levels. The low beta carotene group had five to seven times the risk of getting cataracts. Being an antioxidant it should share with ascorbic acid and vitamin E the ability to be therapeutic for any disease characterized by excess formation of free radicals.

Vitamin A is also known as the anti-infective and anti-opthamalic vitamin. It is important for retention of normal vision, permitting formation of visual purple in the eye, counteracting night-blindness and weak vision. It maintains healthy mucous in the respiratory system and thus fights off infection and allergic symptoms. Vitamin A also promotes protective sheathing around the nerve fibers, tissues, and organs internally and promotes healthy skin, hair and nails.

MINERALS

❧

All life originated in the seas, a vast solution of all the minerals known, mostly in very minute concentrations. Life adapted these minerals to its own needs, utilizing some which became essential and trying to keep many out to the maximum degree possible. Without these minerals there can be no life. And as with vitamins and other nutrients, for each mineral there is an optimum requirement. Too little will inhibit many important reactions in the body and too much will be toxic. For most minerals the useful range is much narrower than it is for vitamins and for some it is very narrow indeed. For some minerals 350 g per day are needed, for others 2–5 mg is the ideal dose, for still others less than 1 mg. Thus minerals cannot be used with the same degree of freedom as vitamins. I have divided the key minerals into categories of absolutely essential, possibly essential, and non-essential.

> *And as with vitamins and other nutrients, for each mineral there is an optimum requirement. Too little will inhibit many important reactions in the body and too much will be toxic.*

LAW

ABSOLUTELY ESSENTIAL

Sodium and Potassium

I will discuss these two minerals together since they have to be in balance. About 4 g of each is required but this varies

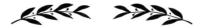

tremendously with a large number of factors. Both elements are involved in the transfer of energy in the body. Sodium remains in the fluid outside the cells, while potassium is held inside the cells. It requires work on the part of the cells to maintain this difference. Unprocessed foods contain much more potassium than they do sodium, but during processing salt is added and this reverses the ratio.

The ratio of potassium over sodium is related to the development of hypertension or high blood pressure. This ratio is call the "K" factor and is determined by measuring the amount of sodium and potassium in the urine. Hypertension affects one out of three people in the United States and in Canada. People with high blood pressure run the risk of dying from stroke, heart failure, or kidney disease. However, while it is developing, they will feel normal. There are some drugs which will decrease the pressure but they carry the risk of side effects. Most of the patients I see who are already taking blood pressure pills do not like the side effects and are keen to come off them.

Blood pressure is considered high if the systolic (the upper reading) is over 140 and the diastolic (the lower) is over 80. It does increase with age and there is a question whether too many people are placed on medication unnecessarily. The old rule was that the systolic should not be higher than 100 plus the age — that is, if a person age 80 had a systolic pressure over 180 he was considered normal, whereas now this would be too high. R.D. Moore and G.D. Webb in their book *The K Factor* concluded that high blood pressure arose from eating too little potassium (in some people too little magnesium or calcium) and too much sodium. Other factors affecting blood pressure are too little exercise and too much weight. In their book, they outline the four basic rules for maintaining normal blood pressure with a detailed description of each. (1) See your doctor. (2) Eat right. Their description of the right diet is exactly what I have been recommending as the orthomolecular diet, the

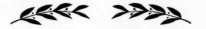

diet our ancestors were forced to eat. For Moore and Webb, "the diet of our remote ancestors may be a reference standard for modern human nutrition and a model for defense against certain 'diseases of civilization'." (3) Exercise. (4) Maintain normal weight.

Magnesium and calcium also play a role in high blood pressure, while the direct role of sodium appears to be less important. The sodium chloride molecule appears to be more of a villain since sodium ion alone is not that bad. The sodium in sodium ascorbate does not pose any risk. It may be that with the right K ratio, increases in sodium are not as dangerous. In one study giving sodium chloride increased systolic and diastolic pressure, whereas giving sodium citrate did not. In one study a series of patients on hypertensive medication were given 1 gram of calcium daily. After a few months half of them no longer needed their medication. With respect to magnesium in areas where the drinking water is low in magnesium there is a higher incidence of high blood pressure. Magnesium salts decrease elevated blood pressure. A study on 21,000 people showed a strong correlation between calcium intake and hypertension. It was the only nutrient which showed this high relationship.

Cerebral hemorrhage (apoplexy) is the second most common cause of stroke. The two most likely precursors are hypertension and abnormalities of the blood vessels. The factors involved in stroke are psychosocial, physiological, and nutritional, namely a deficiency of vitamin C, high salt diets, deficiency of potassium, deficiency of magnesium, deficiency of selenium, excessive lead ingestion, and very low cholesterol levels. Of all these nutritional factors, the most important single factor was a deficiency of magnesium. Five lines of evidence support this view, as H.D. Foster explains in his study *Health, Disease and the Environment*. (1) Global mortality rates. Japan suffers from a very high incidence of stroke. Their soils and drinking water are very low in both calcium and magnesium. The Japanese also tend to

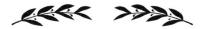

have lower cholesterol levels because their intake of animal products and sugar is much lower. The combination of low cholesterol and low magnesium may be the cause. As the Japanese increase their intake of animal foods their cholesterol levels have risen and the incidence of stroke has fallen 60 percent between 1964 and 1983. Thailand and Egypt have the lowest stroke mortality rate. Their soils and drinking water are very rich in calcium and magnesium. Magnesium intake is particularly high. In the United States and in Britain, areas characterized by high calcium and magnesium intake have a lower incidence of stroke than areas where these minerals are deficient. (2) Declining stroke mortality in the developed world. This is due to the decrease in high cholesterol levels these people have been trying to achieve. There is also a decrease in the consumption of salt. (3) Gender factor. Men have more strokes because they loose magnesium faster than women. Also alcohol increases loss of magnesium. (4) Stroke increases with age. This is true in western countries with the high-tech diets. Diets of the elderly are much more prone to be magnesium deficient. (5) Strokes are more common in the winter. Magnesium is most often much less available in the winter, both in the drinking water and due to the decreased intake of fresh fruits and vegetables. Foster make the useful suggestion that magnesium ought to be added to widely used foods as is being done in Finland. In Finland they are adding potassium and magnesium to salt. This decreases the sodium chloride to 65 percent of the mixture. There is already a decline in mean blood pressure in the study population.

> *The prudent diet to prevent stroke arising from high blood pressure and other causes is to consume a lot less salt, a lot more potassium (more vegetables and fruit and if necessary potassium supplements), a lot more magnesium and more calcium, a lot more vitamin C, a lot less sugar — in short, the orthomolecular diet, the diet to which we have been adapted.*

LAW

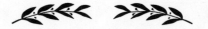

The prudent diet to prevent stroke arising from high blood pressure and other causes is to consume a lot less salt, a lot more potassium (more vegetables and fruit and if necessary potassium supplements), a lot more magnesium and more calcium, a lot more vitamin C, a lot less sugar — in short, the orthomolecular diet, the diet to which we have been adapted. If the cholesterol is elevated and will not come down by diet alone, then nicotinic acid will bring it down. Contrary to medical belief, nicotinic acid is not only a hypocholesterolemic substance, it also elevates the cholesterol if it is too low, by increasing high density lipo protein cholesterol. This provides an additional anti-stroke factor by elevating too low cholesterol levels.

Calcium and Magnesium

Ninety-nine percent of the calcium in our body is in our bones and teeth. Each day 700 mg exchanges between bones and the rest of the body. The remaining one percent is very important in controlling many reactions, such as clotting, muscle function, nerve conduction, cell-wall permeability, and enzyme activity. Only about 25 percent of the calcium in food is absorbed. Absorption is increased by vitamin D, protein, lactose, and an acid medium. High phosphorus levels decrease its absorption, as does phytic acid, oxalate, and fiber. It is also decreased by excess fat, by alkalinity, and by stress. The same amount is absorbed from all the calcium supplements. Preparations which contain more calcium per unit weight are therefore preferable. Adults need about 500 to 1000 mg daily while pregnant and lactating women need about 1500 mg. Milk products provide calcium. Two servings of dairy products will provide about 600 mg of calcium. Those who are dairy allergic will need to take supplements.

A deficiency of calcium is related to osteoporosis, but not directly and an excess to the formation of kidney stones. Osteoporosis is the major disease linked to calcium. The most visible expression is the "dowagers hump." But this disease

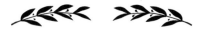

affects many others, between 15 to 20 million adults in North America. Of these, 1.3 million suffer fractures early. The bones are weakened by a decrease in the amount of calcium. Bone mass loss is complicated, depending upon age, sex, race, hormones, nutrition, and activity. The general hypothesis is that bone loss is due to loss of estrogens after menopause, to a deficiency of calcium, and to a deficiency of fluoride. Other deficiencies are manganese, copper, zinc, and boron. Normal bone contains 150 mg per gram of calcium. Osteoporotic bone only 114 mg. It also contains one quarter of the manganese levels found in normal bone. Protein intake has been overlooked as a factor. It was been found that osteoporosis is more common in populations which consume very high protein diets and is much less common in populations which consume low protein diets. Apparently the increased intake of protein demands more calcium and this is withdrawn from the bones. Too much protein increases the loss of calcium in the urine. The ratio of phosphorus to calcium also determines what happens to calcium in bones and in the body. The high-tech diet is very rich in phosphorus which comes from animal protein, soft drinks, preserved foods, food additives, and more. The optimum ratio is about 1:1. Animal protein has a ratio of 26:1, phosphorus over calcium. This disturbed ratio causes loss of bone calcium. The Chinese eat much less animal protein, much more vegetable protein, ingest about 500 mg of calcium daily, and do not have osteoporosis as a major problem.

Recent reviews of the research literature suggest that a combination of calcium and vitamin D will reduce the ravages of osteoporosis. Dr. R. Heaney states that we know enough now to ensure that calcium and vitamin D are used to protect against this disease. Out of 43 studies on calcium intake and bone strength, 26 were positive and 16 were negative. In several studies, giving menopausal women 1000 mg of calcium daily reduced bone loss by one third to one half. In another study, these two supplements decreased non-vertebral

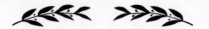

fractures by 32 percent and hip fractures by 43 percent. A 20 percent reduction in hip fractures in U.S.A. would prevent about 45,000 hip fractures and save about $1.5 billion dollars in health costs.

A.R. Gaby and J.V. Wright in their book *Nutrients and Bone Health* describe the following compounds that are or could be used in treating osteoporosis:

1. Estrogens and calcium. These are only partially helpful.
2. An orthomolecular diet. This will not contain excess phosphorus.
3. Vitamin K. This is needed to make osteocalcin, found primarily in bone. The dose ranges from 5 to 10 mg daily.
4. Vitamin D_3. This must be given under medical supervision.
5. Magnesium. The optimum dosage is 250 to 750 mg daily.
6. Manganese. The optimum dosage is 15 to 50 mg daily.
7. Folic acid. The menopause is associated with folic acid deficiency. The optimum dosage is 5 to 15 mg daily. In Canada a prescription is required.
8. Boron. The optimum dosage is 3 to 6 mg daily.
9. Strontium.
10. Silicon.
1.1 Vitamin B-6. A deficiency of this vitamin produced osteoporosis in rats. The optimum dosage is 250 to 500 mg daily.
12. Zinc. The optimum dosage is 25 to 50 mg daily.
13. Copper. The optimum dosage is 1 mg daily.
14. Ascorbic acid. The optimum levels, sublaxative, are 1 to 20 grams daily.

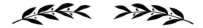

There are other factors as well. Exercise is very important. Weight bearing also is good for the spinal column. Very heavy people do not get osteoporosis as often. When walking it might be a good idea to carry a five pound item to increase the load on the back.

The orthomolecular diet described in this book will prevent most cases of osteoporosis. Treatment should include a normal diet not too rich in protein, optimum amounts of all the trace elements, enough calcium and magnesium. But there is no advantage in gorging on calcium rich foods. Calcium rich foods are milk and cheese. The following quantities should be used: calcium 1-2 grams, magnesium 500 to 1000 mg, zinc 10 to 50 mg, manganese 15-40 mg, boron 3 mg, copper 1-2 mg all daily. I do not recommend fluoride since the best controlled studies have shown it has not had any therapeutic value and may be toxic. However, a recent report by H.D. Foster adds additional evidence in favor of using fluoride. Fluoride is a natural antagonist to aluminum. Indeed it has been found that from one area in South Carolina which had the highest fluoride level in their water the admission rate for Alzheimers was only one fifth what it was from the area with the lowest amount of fluoride in their water. This and other epidemiological evidence lead to the conclusion that "because fluoride reduces the body's absorption of aluminum, it therefore reduces the risk of developing this form of dementia." The same relationship has been found between calcium in the water and Alzheimers. Foster concludes that "if the only significant gain from water fluoridation is reduced tooth decay in children, risks from fluoridation would seem to outweigh gains. However, if as suggested by the evidence presented in this article, because

The orthomolecular diet described in this book will prevent most cases of osteoporosis. Treatment should include a normal diet not too rich in protein, optimum amounts of all the trace elements, enough calcium and magnesium. But there is no advantage in gorging on calcium rich foods.

LAW

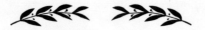

of its antagonism with both aluminum and calcium, moderate levels of drinking water fluoride are protective against Alzheimers disease, osteoporosis and calcification of the arterial system, then the reverse may be true. Obviously, the great fluoridation debate can be expected to continue in earnest."
As well, adequate vitamin D-3 should be obtained. The best sources are the fish oils, cod liver oil and halibut liver oil capsules.

A number of calcium preparations are available. The best are the calcium magnesium complexes providing a ratio of 1:2 or 1:1 of calcium to magnesium. About the same amount of calcium is absorbed from all the available sources. There has been some worry about lead in dolomite. In Canada this is not a factor since quality control is good. About 6 mcg of lead has been found per tablet. But the daily food provides about 300 mcg daily. And since calcium decreases the absorption of lead, it probably adds nothing to the lead burden and may even decrease it. I do recommend dolomite as an inexpensive preparation. The calcium magnesium (Cal-Mag) preparations are preferred over simple calcium salts.

The body contains about 20 to 30 grams of magnesium, half in the bones. The average diet contains about 150 mg per day, which is below the recommended dose. This is due to low magnesium in soils, in water, and in food due to processing. It is the mineral component of chlorophyll. About one third of the magnesium is absorbed. There is an inverse absorption. If calcium is high, less magnesium is absorbed, and if magnesium is high, less calcium is absorbed. Common reasons for too little magnesium are alcoholism, uncontrolled diabetes, excessive use of diuretics, and malabsorption syndromes.

There is no characteristic magnesium deficiency syndrome. The earliest symptoms are loss of appetite, nausea and vomiting, diarrhea, and mental changes. Hyper irritability is common. It should be suspected if there is a potassium

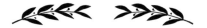

deficiency. Magnesium plays a role in controlling growth of cells and may be useful in treating cancer. Green vegetables are usually recommended by alternative cancer treatments and they are high in magnesium in the chlorophyll. It is also involved in controlling blood pressure. Rats on magnesium deficient diets suffer an increase in blood pressure. Dr. D. McCarron, Division of Nephrology and Hypertension, Oregon Health Services has stated that "for too long we've assumed that the problems with blood pressure in humans are related to an excess of something. . . . Salt has been the culprit nailed repeatedly. But we are frankly amazed at how poor the data base is that links sodium intake to blood pressure." Dr. McCarron concluded that a deficiency of calcium was much more important. He recommends a ratio of calcium to magnesium of 2:1. Other authors recommend a ratio of 1:1. The orthomolecular diet will provide over 500 mg of calcium. Supplements can be used to bring it up to 1000 mg and the magnesium up to 500 to 1000 mg.

The normal diet will provide enough magnesium for most people. When supplements are needed, they should be balanced with calcium, already described. Magnesium in excess will cause diarrhea (thus the use of Epsom salts, high in magnesium, as a laxative). A common preparation is magnesium oxide 420 mg in size.

Iron

The average adult has 3 to 4 g of iron, of which 70 percent is in the hemoglobin. Red cells are recycled every 120 days. Iron is available from food from which 10 percent is absorbed, 30 percent from meat. Absorption depends upon the amount in the food, on vitamin C levels, and on the amount of calcium. It is inhibited by phosphates, phytate, oxalate, and by EDTA, a substance used as a preservative. It may be deficient in cases of malabsorption and after gastrectomy. About one quarter of the female population is deficient. Women lose 50 percent as much iron as men. In men

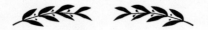

there is danger of too much iron which can cause hemochromatosis. Iron deficiency causes anemia, which is easily diagnosed. On the average men need about 10 mg daily and women about 20 mg during the child bearing years.

Iron is one nutrient that is not used in large doses by orthomolecular physicians. It is difficult to get rid of, and in conditions where there is too much, the patient may have to be bled to get rid of the extra amount. Several years ago there was a vigorous debate over iron supplements when the U.S. Food and Drug Administration wanted to increase the amount of iron filings in flour to decrease the incidence of iron deficiency anemia. Some physicians were already concerned by the over abundance of iron in flour. Luckily it is unlikely any appreciable amount of the iron fillings gets absorbed. It can also be removed by chelating it out with desferoxamine given intramuscularly.

Iron increases the formation of free radicals in the body. Very recently it has been implicated in the pathology of heart disease. Dr. Salonen at the University of Kuopi, Finland, reported that high doses of dietary iron were associated with an increased risk of heart disease. Men with high ferritin levels, the best single measure of stored iron, over 200 mcg per liter were more than twice as likely to have heart attacks. Usually iron overload is diagnosed when levels are over 400 mcg. Dr. Jerome L. Sullivan first proposed there was such a relationship after he observed that iron levels and heart disease risks rose with age in an identical pattern, but his hypothesis and research were rejected by the medical community until recently. The Finnish study has provided powerful support to Sullivan's hypothesis. Dr. Sullivan has argued that the level of iron may turn out to be a more important risk factor than cholesterol or blood pressure levels. It could explain why women are safe from coronary disease until they stop menstruating and can accumulate iron, why oral contraceptives increase the risk because they decrease menstrual blood flow. Jack Challem raised the possibility that it was not

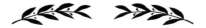

the overload of iron but the deficiency of vitamin E which may have been the main factor. Vitamin E quenches free radicals and could overcome the deleterious effect of iron in increasing them. It is likely both factors are involved. It is prudent to prevent iron overload and also to take enough vitamin E.

Iron overload will also cause mental disease. Cutler reported that iron overload has produced both neurological and psychiatric symptoms in patients with hemochromatosis. He began to look for iron overload in psychiatric patients resistant to treatment. He found seven who showed evidence clinically for overload. They were given twice weekly injections of deferoxamine, 10 mg per kg, i.m. until iron values became normal. There was significant improvement in anxiety, depression, obsessions, compulsions, and panic attacks.

Many people treat themselves with extra iron when they are tired. There is the common belief that fatigue is often caused by anemia. It would be wise not to take any extra iron unless it has been shown that iron deficiency is present. There is a very narrow optimum range for iron therapy.

Zinc and Copper

These minerals are best considered together since there is an inverse connection as measured by serum levels. Most of the 2-3 grams in the body is stored in the bones with a slow turnover. Serum levels range between 80 to 120 mcg. Zinc is one of the most important minerals. Deficiency is very common because it has been dissolved (leached) out of soils, has been removed by centuries of cropping, is removed from grains by processing, dissolves in cooking water, and is removed by chelating agents such as EDTA added to food.

Zinc deficiency causes a large number of symptoms, including stria, stretch marks in both men and women, retarded growth of skin appendages, white areas in the nails, and acne. It interferes with the menstrual cycle (premenstrual

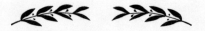

tension), increases blood pressure, causes joint pain, retards wound healing, causes loss of taste and smell, psychiatric symptoms, and acrodermatitis enteropathica. A zinc deficiency is probably present if the subject finds a zinc sulfate solution, which ought normally to taste bitter, to have little or no taste at all. Dr. C.C. Pfeiffer has carried out the best research relating zinc and copper to human health and disease. I have found his book *Zinc and Other Micro-Nutrients* extremely valuable in deciding whether patients should be given extra zinc.

Serum zinc levels tend to be very stable. A large series of patients I analyzed for the presence of copper and zinc showed that with increasing age there was no change in zinc levels whereas copper levels went up significantly after age 50. Recently I saw a patient, age 88, who has been coming to see me every year or two. I saw her first in 1986 when she complained she had lost her sense of taste, that food tasted awful, that she could not smell properly. She found eating almost intolerable but knew she had to. She had been to see nearly 10 physicians, none of whom had been able to help her. I suspected she had a zinc deficiency and started her on zinc supplements using zinc sulfate 220 mg daily. After two years she was no better. One day I asked her why she was still coming since I had not been of any use to her. I secretly hoped she would take that as a hint and not come again because I felt guilty when ever I saw her. She replied that at least I was willing to try to help. At this time I gave her a liquid zinc and manganese preparation developed by Dr. C.C. Pfeiffer (10 percent zinc sulfate and .5 percent manganese chloride). Two years later she was much better. For the past three years she has been well. She told me that she enjoyed eating. One of her new problems was she was a little too heavy. She was cheerful and relaxed and was still on the zinc manganese preparation.

Zinc deficiency is associated with eating disorders. Dr. Schauss summarized the research since 1934 which established a relationship between zinc deficiency and eating

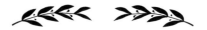

disorders — obesity, pica, anorexia nervosa, and bulimia nervosa. Between 1985 and 1990 several studies showed that most eating disorder patients are low in zinc, and that when they are supplemented with liquid zinc 25 to 110 mg daily, they get better. Occasionally they had nausea which was controlled by pre-treating them with vitamin B-6. Dr. Pfeiffer found that the combination of B-6 and zinc was more efficacious than either one alone. Rita Bakan, a psychologist at St. Paul's Hospital in Vancouver, found that adding zinc to the diet of anorexia patients helped them to regain weight. Vegetarians are more apt to be anorexic and they are also more often low in zinc.

I find the connection between zinc and vitamin B-6 very interesting since it originated in some of our research in Saskatchewan completed 35 years ago. We discovered a mauve staining substance in the urine of most schizophrenic patients when they were sick. If they recovered or went into remission, it disappeared from the urine. This was identified as kryptopyrrole. Dr. Pfeiffer and his group at the Brain-bio center in Princeton discovered that too much of this compound caused a double deficiency of vitamin B-6 and zinc. This condition we had called malvaria, they termed, more appropriately, pyrolleuria. The treatment included ample quantities of zinc and vitamin B-6. While most schizophrenic patients have this factor, it is also present in a smaller proportion of non-schizophrenic patients suffering from depression, anxiety states, alcoholism, and behavioral disorders. It may be present in patients with eating disorders as well. I have described this in the section under vitamin B-6.

In Harrison's *Principles of Medicine,* an inherited zinc deficiency disease called epidermolysis bullosa is described. The symptoms and signs include severe chronic diarrhea, muscle wasting, alopecia, rough thick ulcerated skin about the body orifices and on the extremities. Recently I was consulted by a young man and his mother for help in the treatment of his severe intractable case of epidermolysis bullosa.

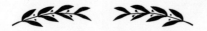

His disease and his response to administration of zinc and a few other nutrients raises the possibility that his condition is a variant of a chronic zinc dependency.

A few days after this patient was born, in June 1972, his skin, which had been under pressure from a forceps delivery, began to slough of. A few days later lesions developed on his face, mouth, chest, and limbs, which later blistered. He was treated with topical antibiotics using sterile technique but was no better. The lesions in his mouth made it impossible for him to feed, and he became anemic and hypoproteinemic. One month later he was diagnosed with epidermolysis bullosa and started on vitamin E 600 i.u. daily, later increased to 800 i.u. At age 4 months 200 mg of ascorbic acid was added, and at age 6 months he was given iron supplementation and the vitamin E was increased to 1000 i.u. There was no response.

He was then admitted to hospital suffering from stomatitis, and again in April 1973 for gastroenteritis and pneumonia. By now he had multiple lesions and denuded areas on his legs, no nails and adhesions between his fingers and his toes. On top of these lesions he had been constantly constipated. His mother had to remove his stools manually daily.

In 1980 his parents took him to West Germany for two and one half months to be treated by a biochemist who was using special skin salves and other treatment, with some success. He was placed upon a vegetarian diet supplemented with a moderate vitamin program, doses unknown. This regimen was helpful. They went back to Germany once more for 10 days and would have gone again but they could no longer afford to do so.

When I first saw him he appeared to be about 10 years old, very short and immature. Mentally he was normal; there were no perceptual changes, no thought disorder, and his mood was surprisingly cheerful and upbeat. The bullous lesions continued to erupt. He had lost all of his fingers and his toes. An attempt had been made to separate them

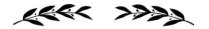

surgically in Italy with no success. He told me that food did not taste normal. He was still severely constipated.

To test his sense of taste for a possible zinc deficiency, I gave him a teaspoon of a special zinc sulfate solution. He said it tasted like stale water, not bitter as it would to normal individuals. I could not order a blood test for zinc since all his superficial veins were gone and it would have required a cut down. Zinc deficiency will cause Dwarfism, retarded wound healing, and loss of taste.

I advised him to start on the following supplements: niacinamide 500 mg bid, ascorbic acid 500 mg tid, pyridoxine 100 mg bid, cod liver oil .5 teaspoon daily, and 10 drops twice each day of a solution of zinc sulfate 10 percent and manganese chloride .5 percent, plus 1 teaspoon of linseed oil daily to increase his intake of omega-three essential fatty acids. Two weeks later he was much improved. His mood remained normal but his parents were much more cheerful. In that brief period he had grown half of an inch in height, his skin was much healthier, and the lesions came on about one third as frequently. Those that did develop healed much more quickly. He gained two pounds and was no longer constipated — he was able to have normal bowel movements for the first time in his life

When I first saw him his mother informed me that he was very sensitive to any tablets. I therefore had him start one nutrient at a time, and if there was no bad reaction, he was to proceed to the next. He had no bad reactions to any of the supplements. I increased his niacinamide to 500 mg tid and the ascorbic acid to 1 gram bid.

This patient's rapid response does not prove it was due entirely to the administration of the zinc. The other nutrients must also have played an important part, but I suspect that zinc was the main therapeutic variable. Single nutrient deficiencies are very rare. I could not in good conscience withhold the other nutrients since I was not certain that one alone might help. This can be determined later on by withdrawing

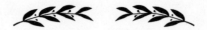

one at a time to determine which are the most important. This family had already suffered too much and needed relief as quickly as possible.

Zinc is water soluble and safe. It is very difficult to overdose but there is no need to do so. Zinc sulfate doses of 220 mg taken three times per day have been recommended for arthritis but usually doses one third that level are sufficient. Dr. C. Pfeiffer described the case of a 16-year-old boy who took 12000 mg over a two day period. He was drowsy for the next week, then recovered. If high doses are taken for too long, it may drive copper levels too far down. This could be a major problem in areas where copper deficiency tends to be common. It is not a problem in Victoria, British Columbia, where I live, for the water is soft and extracts copper from the plumbing in the average home. It is available in various tablets, such as gluconate, sulfate, citrate, and picolinate. There are also zinc chelates. Only a small percentage of the amount taken by mouth is absorbed. Liquid preparations are probably the most easily absorbed. Zinc lozenges are used to ward off the common cold and may be quite effective. Dr. J.C. Godfrey and Dr. B. Conant Sloane at Dartmouth College Health Service compared placebo against a zinc gluconate-glycine preparation for treating the common cold in a double blind study using 23.7 mg of zinc. All symptoms disappeared in 4.9 days against the placebo 6.1 days. If treatment started after one day of the onset, the difference was greater, 4.3 days for the zinc group and 9.2 for the placebo control.

Copper is needed for the formation of hemoglobin. The body contains about 125 mg. On the average we ingest 3 to 5 mg but we need only about 2 mg, so there is some accumulation. Dr. C.C. Pfeiffer found no cases of deficiency in 20,000 patients examined. Many vitamin and mineral preparations contain copper because of the widespread belief that copper deficiency is a serious problem. In certain areas where copper in soil is deficient and babies are fed cow milk,

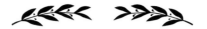

a copper deficiency may develop. Copper tends to accumulate if the diet is too low in zinc or where there is too much copper in the drinking water, usually due to copper plumbing and very soft water. But the danger from too much is much greater. Dr. Pfeiffer considers it to be a toxic element. Excess copper is associated with pregnancy problems, post partum psychosis, depression from birth control pills, and cancer. The best measure of the copper and zinc status is the ratio of serum copper over zinc. The ratio is very high in cancer patients, and high ratios are associated with poor prognosis. Cancer patients with ratios under 1.75:1 have a much better outlook than when the ratio is higher. It has been suggested that the high ratio is also diagnostic. If there is a shadow in the lungs and the ratio is over 1.75:1, it is cancer with a 90 percent probability of being correct. If the ratio is under 1.75, it is probably not cancer.

Dr. Pfeiffer listed eight conditions where copper excess and zinc deficiency would occur: (1) during pregnancy, when growth and development require zinc; (2) during the first year when the newborn has excess copper and needs zinc to balance it; (3) during rapid growth; (4) from the 12th year when the maturing child needs zinc for normal pubertal growth; (5) during teens (if zinc is low, premenstrual tension is common); (6) ages 15 to 20 for stress in general; (7) with stress in adults caused by illness such as cancer, wounds, burns, hypertension, and in senile patients. Excess copper is also associated with a schizophrenic syndrome and with senility. I have found that copper levels increase substantially with age, and that presenile and senile patients have the greatest increase. Excess copper is treated by increasing the intake of zinc using Pfeiffer's solution, Zeman drops (10 percent zinc sulfate and $1/2$ percent manganese chloride), ascorbic acid, high fiber diets, selenium, and, if necessary, copper chelators such as penicillamine and EDTA. Excess levels will be detected by dietary history, by blood tests, and by hair analysis.

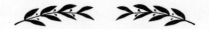

Manganese

The body contains 10 to 20 mg of manganese. About 45 percent is absorbed from food and 4 mg daily is excreted. The diet provides 2 to 9 mg. Manganese deficiency is associated with growth impairment, abnormalities in bone, diabetic-like carbohydrate changes, incoordination, tardive dyskinesia, and convulsions. Zinc alone increases copper excretion in schizophrenics threefold; adding manganese increases the excretion even more. Giving zinc alone may induce a manganese deficiency.

Tranquilizers create a major toxic reaction called tardive dyskinesia, a motor disorder which can be irreversible. About 25 percent of patients on tranquilizers long enough will suffer this disorder. The tranquilizers bind the manganese and are excreted, carrying the manganese with them and so cause a deficiency. Patients I have treated since 1955 with an orthomolecular diet do not get this dreadful condition. Doses up to 30 mg are safe but are seldom needed. I usually use less than 50 mg doses. If the drug companies would put 1 mg of manganese into every tranquilizer tablet, tardive dyskinesia would disappear. I have recommended this to one company but nothing has been done about it. Good natural sources are tropical fruits and tea. British schizophrenics seem not to get tardive dyskinesia as often as America patients, perhaps because they drink much more tea.

Chromium

Glucose tolerance factor (GTF) contains one atom of chromium and two atoms of nicotinic acid. Its structure is not known yet and it may be a family of similar compounds. Dr. Walter Mertz suggested that it was a trivalent chromium atom attached to two niacin molecules and to four amino acids, glutamic acid, cysteine, and glycine. It is an essential cofactor in the activity of insulin. It is thought to attach onto insulin and fasten it on the receptor. Chromium deficiency is more likely than excess since it is present in the part of the

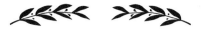

grains commonly not used for food. Whole wheat contains about 1.7 mcg per gram while white flour has only 0.14 ncg. The best sources are brewers yeast, sugar beet molasses, and meats such as liver and beef. Simple chromium salts do not have the same biological activity as GTF chromium. The biological form is absorbed better in the bowel and is more potent as an insulin potentiator, is better for improving impaired glucose tolerance, and is less toxic. Chromium polynicotinate (also called chromium nicotinate) is similar in properties to GTF. The RDA is around 100 mcg daily but the average diet provides only 25 mcg. The body loses more chromium when exercising and when consuming large amounts of sugar.

Chromium in doses of 200 to 400 mcg daily has the following beneficial effects: (1) decreases blood sugar; (2) lowers cholesterol levels and elevates HDL; (3) causes weight loss independent of exercise; and (4) decreases body fat and increased lean body mass. It may be beneficial in preventing coronary disease. It decreases in tissues with age in societies where cardiovascular disease is very common. Given to rats it prevented the formation of atheromatous lesions and increased life span. Chromium potentiated the hypocholesterolemic effect of nicotinic acid, and both taken together in small amounts improved glucose tolerance in elderly subjects, whereas either one alone had no effect. Given to rats it increased their life span by one year or 33 percent.

Selenium

Once considered highly toxic, selenium is now known to be essential. About 200 mcg per day is recommended. When I was working on my M.S.A. in chemistry, I first studied selenium as a toxic component of wheat grown in South Dakota and in southwest Saskatchewan. For awhile there was some apprehension that wheat grown in these areas would be toxic to people. It was soon realized that wheat grown there, even if very high in selenium, would enter the huge

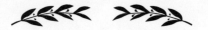

main stream of wheat and would be diluted to the point it could do no harm. Selenium rich soils are found in the Great Plains and Rocky Mountain states. The Northeast, East, and Northwest of the U.S.A. are very low in selenium as is southern British Columbia and Vancouver Island. On the Island animals must be given selenium or they will not grow and thrive. It has the following properties: (1) promotes growth; (2) protects against mercury, cadmium, arsenic, silver, copper, and other heavy metal poisoning; (3) protects against cancer. Populations living on selenium rich soils have less cancer: southern Vancouver Island, low in selenium and carrying more mercury, has a very high incidence of cancer. In a recent study it was found that people had low selenium levels before they had their myocardial infarction.

Selenium also has antidepressant properties and for many may be preferred to the major antidepressants. Benton and Cook found that subjects receiving 100 mcg of selenium improved mood over a five week period compared to placebo. I have been giving my depressed patients 200 mcg twice each day when they do not want to take drugs and the results have been good. The therapeutic dose is between 200 and 600 mcg daily. Patients have taken up to 2000, but I do not recommend this.

POSSIBLY ESSENTIAL MINERALS

Fluoride

The controversy over the addition of fluoride to the public water supply still rages. The proponents of fluoride maintain that it is an important public health measure for decreasing the number of carious teeth in children, and that the only way to ensure it will be used universally is to place it in our water so we will have no choice. They maintain that it is safe. They add that only crackpots and zealots could be against such an important and safe public health measure. The opponents maintain that the improvement in the teeth

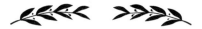

of children is not proven, as the wrong experiments were conducted many years ago, and that there is the same decrease in carious teeth over time in children in areas never fluoridated as well as in fluoridated areas. They also maintain that its safety has not been proven, that, in fact, it is toxic, causing an increase in the incidence of cancer, mottling of teeth, and other undesirable changes. They maintain that if parents want their children to receive the benefit of fluoride, they can use fluoride tooth paste and have their dentists apply it. They are against mass medication of water. They claim that the main reason for the massive use of fluoride today, since it was never established scientifically, was the desire of the chemical companies to dispose of their excess fluoride by dumping it into our drinking water.

The anti-fluoridationists are slowly winning the battle as communities are reversing their stance and making it illegal to use fluoride. *The Medical Tribune* recently carried the headline: "60% of Drinking Water Fluoridated, but Tide Turns." My position is that I would prefer to drink water without fluoride, as I can do in Victoria, that if the public health officials really believe it is so helpful, they should arrange to have two parallel water systems, one for those like me who do not want to be medicated by the public health system and another system for those who do. Those who do want it should pay more, in the same way that anyone wanting medication should bear the increased cost.

Fluoride has been examined as a treatment for osteoporosis. The results of several clinical trials have shown that it is not helpful. There is an increase in bone density but the bones become much more brittle. Dr. Lawrence Riggs at the Mayo Clinic reported the results of a four-year study, in which he gave to 202 postmenopausal women with osteoporosis and vertebral fractures 75 mg of sodium fluoride or placebo. They all received 1,500 mg calcium as well. There was an increase in bone density and a redistribution of bone. Each group suffered the same number of new fractures. But

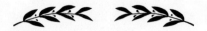

the number of nonvertebral fractures, at the hip, was higher
in the fluoride group. Fluoride users also had more fractures
of the femur. Two thirds of the user suffered severe side
effects. He concluded that fluoride increased bone density
but made the bones too fragile.

NON-ESSENTIAL TOXIC MINERALS

Six metals are toxic — aluminum, mercury, cadmium, silver, gold, and lead. Aluminum is present in our food, in
drinking water, in cooking utensils, in cosmetics, and as a
preservative. Mercury is present in dental amalgams, which
should be called mercury amalgams, not silver amalgams,
since they contain more mercury when they are put in than
silver. Cadmium is present in the air around tires being
worn down by use. Lead was present in gasoline from which
it has been removed but is still present in paint and in some
eating utensils.

I will discuss only aluminum and mercury since both
minerals are the subject of debate between proponents who
maintain they are safe as used and those, like myself, who
maintain that they are toxic and ought not to be used. A similar controversy raged over lead in gasoline. That battle has
been won, but environmentalists and hunters still debate the
effect of lead shot gun pellets and lead sinkers for fishing.
The pellets and weights fall to the bottom of lakes and are
ingested by ducks which are then poisoned by them; in turn,
humans may eat the ducks and be poisoned. There is a
major effort to change the lead pellets to steel or other less
toxic heavy metals. The debate over lead illustrates very
clearly how high-tech societies have approached innovation.
These toxic minerals were added to products because they
added a quality which was desirable commercially. Lead took
out the pinging properties of gasoline. Mercury amalgams
in dental practice are easy to install and aluminum chemicals add certain qualities to food and cosmetics which are

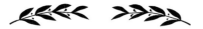

seen to be desirable. When these metals were introduced little thought was given to the effect they would have on the health of the population. After they were used on a large scale, there was a slow, tedious, and costly accumulation of research data showing they were toxic. Finally, after extreme counter pressure, governments, with great reluctance, forced the removal of these products. The procedure seems to be threefold: add the product without concern for the health consequences; prevent any serious examination of the effect on health as long as possible; give way as slowly as possible on the plea that it would be too expensive to change these dangerous practices quickly. Meanwhile millions will have suffered from the exposure to these products.

Aluminum

Organic forms of aluminum are more toxic than aluminum salts. Thus aluminum hydroxide is absorbed poorly from the gut, while aluminum citrate passes rapidly into the blood. The aluminum in drinking water is inorganic and also in salt form. In one study 52 percent was aluminum hydroxide, 29 percent was associated with organic material, and 19 percent was a fluoride complex.

The evidence pointing to aluminum as one of the causes of Alzheimers disease is powerful and becoming stronger. Professor D.R. Crapper McLachlan, Director of the Centre for Research in Neurodegenerative Disease at the University of Toronto, concluded that public health efforts to reduce exposure to aluminum would reduce the incidence of Alzheimers disease. He reviewed four lines of evidence. (1) Aluminum impaired learning and memory performance in animals. (2) Aluminum induced neurochemical changes in the brain. It interferes with over 65 different reactions in the body. It deposits in four sites in the brain — in the neurofibrillary tangles, in the amyloid cores of senile plaques, in the ferritin extracted from the brain, and in the chromatin fractions. Even moderate increases of aluminum in the blood are

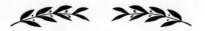

toxic. (3) Many epidemiological studies support the hypothesis. (4) If aluminum is removed using desferoxamine, there is less deterioration compared to a control group. This substance binds aluminum and reduces the amount in the body.

Dr. McLachlan made the following suggestions. Exposure to aluminum should be minimized, but this will be difficult since it is found in food, added to drinking water, many processed foods, cosmetics, toothpaste, and a variety of other cosmetics. Public action is necessary. Aluminum content should be listed on packages and in cosmetic products. Municipal processed water should be regulated so there is less than 50 mcg per liter and eventually less than 10 mcg. Daily intake should be lowered to 3 mg or less.

Mercury

Mercury is a highly toxic liquid mineral with a relatively high vapor pressure which therefore vaporizes very easily. It has been known for many years as a brain toxin which will cause psychosis. The mad hatters of Europe were mercury intoxicated hat makers. Mercury vapor will rarely be a factor today. However, about 20 years ago I saw two men in one month both with the schizophrenic syndrome caused by prolonged contact with liquid mercury. Eliminating the mercury also eliminated the psychotic condition.

The major source of intoxication from mercury comes from our mouths, from the mercury amalgams dentists have introduced. The mercury is thereafter absorbed both from the vapor and from direct contact with tissue in the gums. But this view is stoutly attacked by the dental profession and by the medical profession. The debate is as vigorous over mercury from our amalgams as it was for lead and as it is for fluoride, but it has not yet entered the public arena as have the other two controversies.

Dr. Hal Huggins is one of the early and strongest critics of the use of mercury amalgams. The sharpest scientific attack comes from Dr. Murray J. Vimy, Clinical Professor in

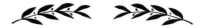

the Department of Medicine, University of Calgary, and Dr. D. Shwartzendruber, Chair of the Biology Department, University of Colorado. Dr. Shartzendruber presented evidence to the Washington State Dental Disciplinary Board which was holding hearings on a proposed restriction regarding dentists making statements against the use of mercury amalgams. He noted that mercury amalgams contain over 50 percent mercury, 35 percent silver, 13 percent tin, and lesser amounts of copper. Contrary to the view put forward by the dental profession, mercury is not harmless when present in the amalgam with other metals since it gradually disappears from the amalgams and seeps into the rest of the body. It is released as vapor which is increased by chewing. The amount released daily accumulates. The mercury lodges in the tissues, is absorbed by the lungs and intestinal tract, and accumulates in the brain and other organs. Methyl mercury is absorbed from the mouth and goes directly to the brain. Shartzendruber added that as a general toxin it affected all tissues. There is no safe level except zero. He concluded that the World Health Organization had determined that amalgams were the prime source of human mercury exposure. In his view people in general looked upon mercury toxicity as close to asbestos and ddt, above lead paint and auto emissions and slightly below PCBs and uranium mining.

Dr. Murray Vimy reported the results of his studies with sheep to the Washington State Dental Disciplinary Board Public Hearing. He placed mercury amalgams in sheep and studied what happened to the mercury. Within 30 days substantial amounts of mercury were taken into their tissues. The same occurred with monkeys. Sheep lost 50 percent of their ability by their kidneys to recycle sodium and a decrease in the secretion of albumen. He then referred to studies which showed that Alzheimer's patients have five to eight times as much mercury in their brains than the normal population. The greatest amount was found in those parts of the brain where the Alzheimers lesions were present.

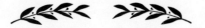

He concluded that mercury is released from amalgams; it is released continuously when we chew; in animal models it is taken up into the tissues, particularly the liver, gastrointestinal tract and kidneys; it can induce pathology in sheep; removal of the mercury improves kidney function; there is a link to Alzheimers disease; there is a link with development of antibiotic resistant bacteria. The board eventually decided not to bring in their pernicious recommendation.

In a recent paper Dr. A. Summers, Professor of Microbiology at the University of Georgia, reported that mercury fillings weakened the effectiveness of antibiotics against bacteria. This means that for some patients the usual amount of antibiotic will be inadequate and they will have to be given much higher doses, and for others the antibiotic will be ineffective at any dose. The implications are chilling. Some bacteria were resistant to six antibiotics.

Recently Dr. Siblerud found that a very significant deterioration of psychological health occurred in people with mercury amalgams and an improvement when these fillings were removed. Fifty subjects with fillings had 1.43 ppm in their hair and 3.70 ppm in urine compared with 50 with no fillings who had 1.13 in hair and 1.23 in urine. The amalgam group were more depressed, had less peace of mind, had more problems in concentration. They had more than twice as many complaints, such as sudden outbursts of anger, depression, irritability, and anxiety. They craved sweets more, smoked more, and drank more coffee and alcohol. A further study on subjects after the mercury was removed showed that 80 percent felt much better. They were less nervous, less depressed, felt more confident, and their memory was better. Recently one of my female patients had all her amalgams removed. She had been depressed for many years and had failed to get well after two years of psychiatric treatment, but within a few weeks after the mercury was removed she was free of depression. Higher levels of lead and mercury have been found in the hair of emotionally disturbed children.

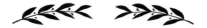

Not everyone will need to have their amalgams removed even though this would be ideal. But whenever a person has any physical or mental problem for which there appears to be no cause and which has remained untreatable, it is important to examine the question whether mercury amalgams might be an important factor. More dentists are familiar with mercury toxicity and have developed methods for helping determine whether there is a problem. They take special precautions not to expose themselves to mercury. Even their associations who stoutly defend the use of mercury advise their members not to be exposed to it. They think it is all right to maintain continuous exposure in one's mouth but not in their offices. Even undertakers now have to be careful. So many bodies being cremated contain mercury there is a great danger that the mercury vapor will injure them while they are working. Dentists will want mercury analysis of blood and urine and will do certain conductivity tests in the mouth plus their personal examination of the teeth. Everyone should insist that mercury amalgams not be used and gradually replace existing mercury amalgam fillings with other material. When the demand for other safer compositions becomes noticeable, the manufacturers will surely meet the demand and dentists will learn the necessary skills with which to work with these materials.

The final diagnosis of metal toxicity for aluminium and mercury as well as for cadmium, silver, gold, and lead is made by laboratory tests, namely blood analysis, urine analysis, and hair analysis. Once toxicity is diagnosed, the source of the toxic mineral must be determined and withdrawn. Then the orthomolecular diet should be instituted. Removing additives decreases the toxic burden on the body and adding fiber increases the excretion of toxic minerals. Then chelating compounds are used. The safest is ascorbic acid which should be given in optimum doses. The three other chelating compounds which bind minerals and remove them are penicillamine for copper, desferoxamine

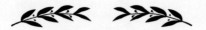

for aluminum and iron, and EDTA for iron and other compounds. This is called chelation therapy when it is given by vein in a series of treatments. Finally one should use natural antidotes such as selenium against mercury and cadmium, zinc and manganese against copper, zinc against cadmium.

AMINO ACIDS AND ESSENTIAL FATTY ACIDS

※

AMINO ACIDS

Eight amino acids are considered essential supplements since they cannot be made in the body and adequate amounts must therefore be present in the food. These include l-tryptophan, phenylalanine, lysine, arginine, ornithine, and tyrosine. The other 14 amino acids are interconvertible in the body and for this reason have not been labeled "essential." These include glutamic acid, aspartic acid, cysteine, methionine, glycine, histidine, alanine, methionine, proline, serine, and threonine. They are all *essential*, however, and if there is a metabolic problem resulting in a deficiency of any of the 22, the results would be devastating to the body. There have been few systematic orthomolecular studies of the non-essential amino acids, but the eight essential amino acids have been examined more carefully and some have found a role in orthomolecular treatment. I will discuss l-tryptophan and tyrosine and phenylalanine from the essential group because they are so similar to each other, and glutamic acid from the non-essential group.

> *Eight amino acids are considered essential supplements since they cannot be made in the body and adequate amounts must therefore be present in the food.*

LAW

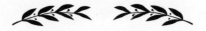

L-tryptophan

Tryptophan is used clinically when it is thought that it will increase the production of serotonin in the brain. Serotonin is probably involved in controlling mood and sleep, with a deficiency causing depression and insomnia. It is also a precursor of vitamin B-3 in the form of nicotinamide adenine dinucleotide (NAD). Most of the tryptophan proceeds down the pathway which leads to NAD but only 1.6 grams from 60 grams is converted to it. Pellagra is caused by a deficiency of tryptophan and vitamin B-3. The usual pellagra producing diet was rich in corn and very deficient in high quality protein containing foods. It had too little tryptophan, too little vitamin B-3, too little isoleucine, and too much leucine.

Tryptophan is used for treating depression as well for controlling manic depressive mood swings. It may be used alone or in combination with other antidepressants, such as the amine oxidase inhibitors, tyrosine and lithium. I have used tryptophan for at least the past 30 years but primarily for patients with insomnia. It is very helpful to 50 percent of the patients and they awaken in the morning without hangover. They much prefer it to hypnotics.

In the United States, tryptophan is not available because many fear it is toxic. Although it has been shown that the toxicity was caused by a contaminant, not by pure amino acid, this amino acid still has not been released and is now the center of a major controversy between the FDA and the health food industry and physicians who had been using it very successfully. In Canada it was available from health food stores and also on prescription. The health food store preparation has been withdrawn but the prescription products called Tryptan has not and has been freely available throughout that controversy.

Here is what happened. In October 1989 several people in New Mexico became very tired with sore muscles. Their white blood cells were increased. All had taken the amino acid. This condition was later called eosinophilia-myalgia

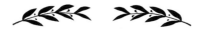

syndrome (EMS) and was reported in Europe and elsewhere in America. Symptoms included pain, swelling of the extremities, and severe muscle symptoms involving nerve damage. The eosinophil count went high. By August 1990 more than 1500 cases had been reported with 27 deaths. In November 1989 tryptophan supplements were recalled, and a few months later all products containing tryptophan were also recalled.

The Center for Disease Control suggested, however, that the problem was caused by a contaminant. Six companies in Japan made all the tryptophan used in the United States. In October 1990 K. Sakimoto isolated and identified an impurity from tryptophan which in acid fluid, like in the stomach, broke down into tryptophan and a toxic chemical. Even though tryptophan was thus proven safe and effective, the FDA has still not removed its ban on its use. The health food industry believes that this is a political decision, not based upon scientific data, and is fighting back.

Tryptophan is used in doses of 500 mg to 12 grams daily. For insomnia, the dose is 1 to 3 grams taken before bed on an empty stomach. If it is taken with food, it has difficulty passing into the brain and therefore has no effect on the serotonin levels. When taken on an empty stomach, it does not have to compete with other amino acids. For depression I have been using 3 to 6 grams daily, as well as for manic depressives (the bipolar disease).

Phenylalanine and Tyrosine

Phenylalanine is partially converted into tyrosine. When the body cannot make any, it causes a condition known as phenylketonuria. Untreated it leads to mental retardation which may be very severe. These children have to be on special phenylalanine free diets. Phenylalanine is used as a treatment for depression; the dl-form is helpful in controlling pain. Tyrosine is a precursor to catecholamines (noradrenalin, etc.) and to thyroid hormone. It is also the precursor to

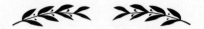

melanin, a major pigment in the body. It has antidepressant properties, probably because it acts in the same way in the body as does phenylalanine.

Dr. Priscilla Slagle, a psychiatrist, uses a combination of tryptophan with phenylalanine and tyrosine as a treatment for depression. She was depressed herself for many years, did not respond to the usual treatment, but recovered on the program she developed, as she describes in her book *The Way Up From Down*. She recommends that people suffering from depression take tyrosine 500 to 3500 mg on rising in the morning and again mid afternoon. These should be taken without high protein food. One starts with 500 to 1000 mg daily for one week, then the dose is increased gradually depending upon the response. After several weeks or months if the response is not adequate, she adds phenylalanine to the program.

She also recommends l-tryptophan, 500 to 6000 mg at bed time, taken on an empty stomach or with carbohydrate, not with protein; B complex (50) at breakfast and again after dinner at night; ascorbic acid, to 4 grams daily; and a good multimineral preparation providing calcium 250-1000 mg, magnesium 125-599 mg, manganese 10-30 mg, zinc 15-30 mg, selenium 50-200 mcg, and chromium 50-200 mcg. Dr. Slagle also prescribes dietary changes to improve this. Everyone who is depressed ought to read her book. The results are probably as good if not better than the results using antidepressant drugs. The program is more complicated than simply taking a few pills each day but for many may be preferable.

In Canada tyrosine and phenylalanine are not readily available. The Food and Drug Division of Health and Welfare appears to want to prevent people from looking after their own health by placing a number of unwarranted restrictions on the sale of amino acids. In 1989 their expert advisory committee on amino acids submitted the results of their deliberations: "low daily doses of the amino acids, such as

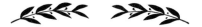

500 mg in capsule form, were perceived as not being harmful for the healthy individual, with the possible exception of tryptophan. There was no evidence that consumption of free-form amino acids in amounts equivalent to the daily intake would be unsafe if added to the daily diet and consumed throughout the day." However, the committee saw no rationale for the use of the amino acids as nutritional supplements and worried about the long term side effects: "there would appear to be no convincing rationale for having amino acids generally available to the public. If amino acids exert the pharmacological effects claimed, they are unsafe if not taken under medical supervision for a specific benefit; if they do not exert these effects, then there is no reason for marketing them. Furthermore, all of these amino acids were considered to have the potential for producing certain toxic effects in susceptible individuals or if consumed in large amounts for an extended duration." The key word is potential. There is nothing which is not potentially dangerous, even water. They did not discuss the actual toxic reactions and harm done to people who had taken these amino acids without medical supervision, or even with it.

On the one hand, the committee concluded these amino acids were safe. On the other hand, they concluded they might be dangerous. The FDD is tied to their pet scheme that anything for which claims are made, except for food, must be dispensed by prescription to protect the public. Since the use of amino acids, like vitamins, cannot be patented, there is no incentive for any company to spend the immense sums of money required to convince the FDD that they should not interfere in the sale of these safe products. If they were to be consistent, all the vitamins must be taken off the market. This, I think, they are afraid to do because of the enormous backlash from the public and even from the medical profession which would be inundated with huge number of patients demanding prescriptions. It would be similar to the experience in the Canadian Maritime provinces long ago when

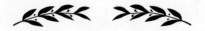

people could buy liquor only on prescription. There have been rumors that they are thinking of such a move but I was advised by one of the ministers of health, when I inquired, that they would never do so. But as few people are aware of the value of the amino acid, they can with impunity introduce regulations which in my opinion are totally unwarranted. They hope that the public remains generally ignorant and that people will never develop the same enthusiasm and affection for amino acids that they now have for vitamins and minerals. They are trying to forestall a problem they see developing which would go against their policies. The FDD should be restricted to making sure that all products sold are non toxic (that is, less toxic than are the over-the-counter drugs they allow all drug stores to dispense so freely) and that the label requirements are met. I would be happier if they would put aspirin on prescription. Many people die from aspirin each year, while no one has died from the use of pure vitamin and amino acid supplements.

In my opinion, Dr. D. Rowland, Canadian Institute of Nutrition made the most sensible recommendation. He argued that the consumer should be allowed access to these nutrients because amino acids are similar to vitamins and hence are non toxic; there are more hazardous substances available, such as cigarettes and alcohol. All of the over-the-counter non-prescription items such as antihistamines, analgesics, cough medicines and more are much more dangerous than any of the nutrients. The consumer should be helped to make informed choices. If no benefit is derived from a product the consumer will not buy it.

> **LAW**
>
> *The consumer should be allowed access to these nutrients because amino acids are similar to vitamins and hence are non toxic; there are more hazardous substances available, such as cigarettes and alcohol.*

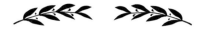

L-glutamine

Glutamine is made from glutamic acid, one of the so-called non-essential amino acids but which is still very essential. Glutamic acid does not pass readily across the blood-brain barrier but glutamine is more successful. Dr. Roger Williams used l-glutamine many years ago to decrease the use of alcohol by rats. Studies with alcoholics showed a similar therapeutic effect. It also decreased craving. There have also been a few studies using glutamic acid and glutamine to enhance I.Q. The dose varies between 500 to 4000 mg per day. Dr. Newbold recommends increasing it slowly.

ESSENTIAL FATTY ACIDS

Over the past 40 years I have seen a marked change in medical opinion of nutrition and the use of nutrients as supplements. In 1950 when I first began to practice medicine, it was generally believed that nutrition played a very minor, if any, role in the practice of medicine. Nutrition was not taught in medical schools, and physicians allowed non clinical nutritionists and dietitians to take over the whole field. In 1955 the first paper was published which introduced the concept that large doses of vitamins could be used therapeutically for treating conditions not known to be vitamin deficiency diseases. The decade 1970 to 1980 marked the beginning of the megavitamin decade. The following decade saw the introduction of mineral supplements on a larger scale. The 1990s could be called the essential fatty acid (EFA) decade.

There has been an enormous rise of interest in these fats and oils, and the roles they play in a large number of diseases. This includes the study of cardiovascular disease and the connection between cholesterol and other fats and a large number of the chronic diseases. EFAs are essential nutrients and play a major role in our health and well-being

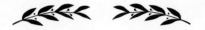

as do essential vitamins, amino acids, and minerals.

The essential fatty acids, omega-3, and omega-6 series, began to disappear from our diet about 75 years ago. Only 20 percent of our needs are available in the average diet today. Dr. D. Rudin and Dr. C. Felix call essential fatty acids the nutritional "missing link." They have presented convincing evidence that this missing nutrient is one of the main factors in producing much of the illness we have to contend with in our modern high-tech society. Omega-3 essential fatty acids are highly reactive fatty acids, some of which are converted in the body into the essential prostaglandins. The other essential series are the omega-6 fatty acids. They must be in balance. They are needed for growth, for many metabolic roles, for the integrity of the cell membranes, and to prevent skin drying and flaking.

> **LAW**
>
> *The decade 1970 to 1980 marked the beginning of the megavitamin decade. The following decade saw the introduction of mineral supplements on a larger scale. The 1990s could be called the essential fatty acid (EFA) decade.*

The common vegetable oils have a lot of the omega-6 fatty acid but are deficient in the omega-3 type. The omega-3 group are chemically more reactive, have lower melting points (they are more liquid at room temperature), and are made in cold climate plants to make them more resistant to freezing. One of the best sources is linseed oil made from flax seed. Linseed oil used to be a very popular and widely consumed oil but now is mostly available in health food stores. It is very rich in omega-3 oils, up to 60 percent. Omega-3 fatty acids are also found in seafood.

The omega-6 essential fatty acids play an equally important role in maintaining health. Dr. David F. Horrobin has been one of the foremost investigators who have brought these essential fatty acids to medical attention. It is made in the body by adding one double (unsaturated) bond to linoleic acid. It is found mainly in plant seeds, notably in

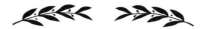

evening primrose, borage, and black currant.

As with all EFAs, the omega-6 series has two main functions: to provide flexibility to cell membranes and control behavior of membrane bound proteins; to control a large number of rapid reactions in the body. EFAs assist the body in making gamma linolenic acid (GLA). Horrobin lists the following conditions which have been helped by GLA: atopic eczema, diabetic neuropathy, premenstrual syndrome, breast pain and prostatic hypertrophy, rheumatoid arthritis and other forms of inflammation, systemic sclerosis, Sjogrens syndrome, and dry eyes associated with contact lenses, gastrointestinal disorders, viral infection and post-viral fatigue syndrome, endometriosis, schizophrenia, alcoholism, cardiovascular disease, renal disease, cancer, and liver disease. It is clear that GLA is not a specific treatment for anything but that it has an enormous importance in the general health of the body. It helps repair biochemical problems which have helped create these pathological diseases. The simplest way of getting GLA is by taking evening primrose oil and other GLA rich oils. The dose range varies from under 1 gram per day to 10 grams for very serious conditions.

Fats and Oils by Udo Erasmus is one of the best simple books that describes the chemistry and biochemistry of the two series of essential fatty acids. In the body EFAs are converted into prostaglandins which help regulate the entire body. When there is a deficiency, digestion is compromised, healing is retarded. There are about 25 important reactions in the body that depend upon having the right amount and kind of prostaglandins. The conversion to prostaglandins requires a large number of cofactors such as vitamins and minerals.

Dr. Rudin and Dr. Felix suggests that pellagra is due to the deficiency of these prostaglandins and that this may occur for two reasons: (1) a deficiency of these cofactors such as vitamin B-3, the best known cause of pellagra; and (2) a deficiency of the essential fatty acids so that even in the presence

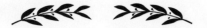

of these cofactors not enough prostaglandins can be made. The first type of pellagra is the cofactor pellagra (vitamin B-3, vitamin B-6, tryptophan) and the second type is a substrate pellagra. The two pellagras are responsible for many of the chronic illnesses, including both mental and physical illnesses.

Here is the oils supplement program recommended by Rudin and Felix:

1. Select the best oil you can. Ideally this is linseed oil. This oil tends to become rancid and develop a very bad flavor. All oils should be tested first. I will discuss this further on. It should be stored cold. Other oils are soybean oil, walnut oil, and wheat germ oil. A 100 pound person can start with 1 tablespoonful of linseed oil daily and a 200 pound person with 3 to 4. It is important not to take more than is needed as the extra oil can cause some side effects.

2. Be sure your diet is vitamin and mineral rich. Magnesium, biotin, zinc, pyridoxine, calcium, and ascorbic acid are needed for normal EFA formation. Vitamin B-3 is needed for the conversion to prostaglandins. Fiber is also very important.

3. Maintain the program by adjusting the amounts. One's health is used as the measure looking at such things as skin texture and feeling of well being. The amount of supplementary oil should be the smallest amount for maintaining good health.

4. Balance the two series, the omega-3 and omega-6. This is done by using both linseed oil and some of the other oils. During the winter season one will need more of the omega-3 and during hot weather less. Fish oils are very good as is evening primrose oil which contains important omega-6 fatty acids.

Obtaining the correct oils is not that simple, however. John Finnegan in his book *The Facts about Fats* discusses some

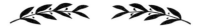

of the problems in the preparation of the commercial oils and fats. If we are to use these essential nutrients with skill and safety, it is important that we understand their chemistry and know how these oils are made. They are very unstable; they have double bonds in them which are avid for oxygen. This is why linseed oil is used to make a base for paint. For the same reason, once the oils have been extracted they will not store very well. During their deterioration or oxidation the oils are changed to products which are of no value and which may be harmful. Manufacturers have tried to avoid some of these changes by using what is called a 'cold' pressing process, which is supposed to avoid the use of heat. Heat increases oxidation and deterioration. But even when the oil is cold pressed, there is a lot of heat generated in the process, unless the oil is pressed so slowly that the heat has a chance to dissipate. This means that the cold pressed oils are little better than the heat treated oils. However, there are a few manufacturers who have produced oils that are very little deteriorated, and they store their oils under nitrogen until the bottle is opened.

Finnegan recommends that high quality oils must be produced by pressing at temperatures under 118° F. using light and oxygen excluding methods, then bottled in containers that prevent exposure to light that causes the oil to go rancid. He also recommends that the oils should be produced from third party, certified organically grown seed.

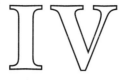

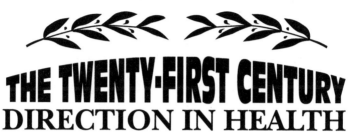

THE TWENTY-FIRST CENTURY
DIRECTION IN HEALTH

ORTHOMOLECULAR PREVENTION AND THERAPY CASE STUDIES

Y

All good food to which anyone has adapted is both preventive and therapeutic. It prevents the diseases which will inevitably occur if the food is deficient in quantity or quality, and if the diet of a person which had made him sick is corrected, it will help restore his health. There is a major exception to this. This is the case where the deficient diet has been the main diet for such a long time that there is permanent damage to the body or to its biochemistry. A combination of severe stress and starvation will lead to permanent impairment of the nutritional biochemistry and only the administration of very large amounts of some of the vitamins will allow that person to function adequately. This is happening now in those countries where there is major starvation, but when it is combined with stress as it is in Africa, with war and brutality, the impact on the population is going to be even worse.

> **LAW**
>
> *All good food to which anyone has adapted is both preventive and therapeutic. It prevents the diseases which will inevitably occur if the food is deficient in quantity or quality, and if the diet of a person which had made him sick is corrected, it will help restore his health.*

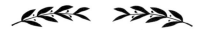

I have already described the effect of an inadequate diet on rats. There was a steady deterioration in their health until the eighth generation after which it remained bad. And this was on a diet that was the same each year. If the diet continues to deteriorate each year, the effect on the health of the animals must be even worse. When they were placed on a good diet, it required four generations to recover their original state of health. It is possible that these rats, if given the right vitamins as supplements, might have regained their health faster.

HONG KONG VETERAN

During the Second World War human population experiments were carried out by the Germans and by the Japanese. I will not discuss the impact of the concentration camps on the survivors except to point out they too became vitamin dependent and responded when they were given large doses of niacin. My experience with the impact of the Japanese experiment came from the Canadian soldiers imprisoned in Hong Kong who came to me for help long after this war was over. The first one was Mr. George Porteous, later Lieutenant Governor of Province of Saskatchewan.

I first met Mr. Porteous when I was doing a study on the effect of niacin upon elderly people living in a nursing home of which he was director. I had explained to him how the people might react to the niacin so that he would be familiar with the flushing effect. He asked me whether he could himself take the niacin. He wanted to experience first hand the flush so that he could be more reassuring to them. About six months later, in the fall of 1960, he came to see me at the University Hospital. He told me that he was a Hong Kong Veteran, that he had been a prisoner of war in a camp in the far east for 44 months. He described the horrible conditions he and the other Canadian soldiers had to endure. It was an extraordinary combination of stress, brutality, and starvation. The death rate was very high. At the end of the war when

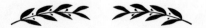

they were liberated, one quarter of the soldiers who had been captured were dead. They all suffered from diarrhea, pellagra, scurvy, beri beri, and almost every nutritional deficiency known.

He described what he was like from his release to the time he began to take the niacin, 3 grams daily. He had lost one third of his body weight. On the hospital ship coming back to Canada, the doctors gave the soldiers the only vitamin supplements they then had, mostly rice bran polishings. Mr. Porteous regained his weight but not his health. From that moment on he was anxious, tense, very sensitive, fearful, physically weak, and suffering from arthritis. He could not lift his arms over his shoulder. He continually consulted the doctors of the Department of Veteran Affairs who treated him with amphetamines in the morning and barbiturates at night to help him sleep. Eventually on the very flimsiest of evidence (hearsay from another person) he was diagnosed neurotic and sent to a psychiatric ward. He came back even worse because his self esteem had dropped even further. He then received sympathetic psychotherapy in Saskatoon and he regained the state he was in before he was admitted to the psychiatric ward. He told me he could not tolerate either heat or cold.

But a month or so after he had started to take the niacin he became normal. All the symptoms vanished. His favorite opening gambit when he saw his family doctor was to stretch his arms to the ceiling and say, "See that." Previously he could not raise them over his shoulders. Mr. Porteous wanted me to know about this miraculous response to niacin. Two years later he went with his son to the mountains for two weeks. He forgot to take with him his niacin. By the time he came home all the symptoms he had suffered previously were coming back. He never forgot to take them thereafter and remained well until his death when he was Lieutenant Governor.

This aroused my interest in the fate of the Hong Kong

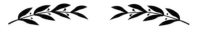

veterans. About 2000 soldiers were freed from the camps but never recovered their health, unlike their siblings who had served in Europe and in other areas during the same war. They continually demanded that something be done for them and eventually the Canadian government appointed a commission which examined their claims for a special pension. The commission found that they were in fact very ill. They had a very high death rate, a high rate of cardiovascular disease, about 25 percent suffered from neurosis, psychoses, and neurological diseases. All the Hong Kong veterans were awarded a special pension.

Mr. Porteous told his fellow POWs about his success with niacin therapy, and within a few years I treated a dozen Canadian vets and some POWs from the United States. Later the information spread to other POWs. Without exception veterans who went onto the vitamin program recovered fully or enough so that they were pleased with their new health. After my experience with the veterans and after reading the literature, I concluded that one year in the camps had aged the veterans by four years. A prisoner in camp four years would come back having aged the equivalent of 16 years. Other investigators had come to a similar conclusion. By this time I was familiar with the concept of vitamin dependency. I have concluded that severe food deprivation combined with stress experienced long enough will cause a vitamin B-3 dependency, and that these individuals will never be well until their increased need for niacin is recognized and they start taking 3 or more grams daily. For these patients made ill by their food, restoring the food is therapeutic, although it may not be enough for those made vitamin dependent. The natural diet is thus both preventative and therapeutic.

> *I have concluded that severe food deprivation combined with stress experienced long enough will cause a vitamin B-3 dependency, and that these individuals will never be well until their increased need for niacin is recognized and they start taking 3 or more grams daily.*

LAW

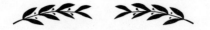

IMPROVED I.Q.

Single nutrients are seldom used for prevention and for treatment, with the exception of niacin which we discovered lowered total cholesterol when it was given alone in large enough doses. It is recognized that on our modern high-tech diets any deficiencies are multiple and involve both vitamins and minerals. This is one reason why the B complex preparations have become so popular and also the vitamin-mineral preparations. Almost all the patients treated by orthomolecular therapists are advised to take more than one vitamin, although it is not necessary to give them individual pills containing these nutrients separately. I will discuss two conditions where multivitamin and multimineral preparations were used and yielded valuable results.

In 1988, David Benton and Gwilym Roberts reported in the British Medical Journal, *The Lancet,* that vitamin and mineral supplements increased intelligence of school children not considered to be nutritionally deprived. Benton and Roberts completed a double blind experiment on 60 children. Thirty were given a vitamin-mineral supplement containing the following: bioflavonoids 50 mg; biotin 100 mcg; choline bitartrate 70 mg; folic acid 100 mcg; inositol 30 mg; niacin 50 mg; pantothenic acid 50 mg; para-aminobenzoic acid 10 mg; pyridoxine 12 mg; thiamin 3.9 mg; riboflavin 5 mg; vitamin A 375 mcg; vitamin B-12 10 mcg; vitamin C 500 mg; vitamin D-3 3 mcg; vitamin E 79 i.u.; vitamin K 100 mcg; calcium gluconate 100 mg; chromium 0.1 mg; magnesium 7.6 mg; manganese 1.5 mg; molybdenum 0.1 mg; iodine 50 mcg; iron 1.3 mg; and zinc 10 mg. Thirty were given placebo.

After eight months there was no significant difference between the groups on verbal intelligence scores. However, only the supplemented group increased non-verbal intelligence scores. Non-verbal I.Q. increased from 111 to 120, while with placebo it remained unchanged at 109. Verbal intelligence is a measure of an individual's unique cultural,

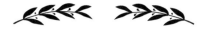

educational, and environmental experiences. Non-verbal intelligence is considered to be innate or biologic in nature; the answers do not require general information and vocabulary. The growth curve of non-verbal intelligence parallels other physical factors such as brain weight. Improved nutrition would be expected to affect non-verbal I.Q. first, but later with the interplay of an enriched environment, verbal I.Q. would also be expected to rise. In a recent report Benton and Cook confirmed their earlier findings on a different population. Intelligence was increased by 7.6 points, while on placebo there was a decline of 1.7 points.

> *These two studies lead to two conclusions: (1) Even normal children on the usual diet are more intelligent after they are given very moderate doses of vitamins and minerals. (2) Mentally retarded children need more vitamins and minerals.* **LAW**

C.F. Harrell *et al* (1981) reported similar findings when mentally retarded children were given vitamins and mineral supplements plus thyroid. This paper stirred up a hornets' nest, so much so that seven attempts have been reported to repeat the Harrell study, yet none of the seven repeated it successfully. However, they used a different type of population of children and did not use thyroid. It seems too difficult for critics to really repeat work of which they are critical.

These two studies lead to two conclusions: (1) Even normal children on the usual diet are more intelligent after they are given very moderate doses of vitamins and minerals. (2) Mentally retarded children need more vitamins and minerals. Over the past 35 years I have treated about 1500 children with vitamins and minerals. I have no doubt that there is a major improvement in their intelligence performances following their recovery. I don't think any one can perform at their best when they are ill, depressed, have poor concentration, or difficulty with memory.

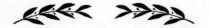

DOWN'S SYNDROME

Down's Syndrome, at one time considered an excellent example of a disease caused by bad mothering, is one of the genetic diseases and therefore considered untreatable by many physicians and psychiatrists. Dr. Henry Turkel was the first physician to think otherwise. He began to treat cases of Down's Syndrome over 40 years ago using a combination of vitamins, minerals, and hormones. He began to see major recoveries among the patients he treated. The parents of the children he treated were very enthusiastic about his treatment, but his views were so outrageous to the establishment that no one paid any attention to him. The FDA tried to suppress his work and eventually he was permitted to treat only patients in his own state of Michigan. He used every technique known to disseminate his views in medical journals, but he was rejected by the editors and their committees. He did have some of his work published in a journal I was editing and more recently he published a book called *Medical Treatment of Down's "Syndrome"*, where he presented individual case histories and photographs of the children before and after treatment. But there appears to be no one in North America who is showing the slightest interest in the amazing results he was able to get. As Professor Linus Pauling comments in his introduction to this book, "The work of Dr. Henry Turkel provides a striking example of the way in which this opposition operates to the detriment of the health and well being of a large number of people. Dr. Turkel has developed, over a period of decades, a treatment of mentally retarded children with the use of vitamins, minerals and cerebral stimulants, and other substances. He has gathered together a convincing body of clinical observations showing the genetic condition of mental retardation need not be accepted as inevitably leading to permanent defect and inability of the individual to function in normal society. Dr. Turkel has indeed provided new hope for the mentally

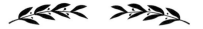

retarded and for members of there families, hope that a great improvement in functioning can be achieved."

In the same book Dr. Bernard Rimland wrote, "Government sponsored research designed to thoroughly evaluate the Turkel treatment should have been started 30 years go. Perhaps, if the readers of this book write to their representatives in Congress in sufficient numbers, such research may yet be done. In the meantime, what of the millions of retarded children whose treatment could have begun years ago but for FDA opposition? . . . The thought is appalling. If I were the parent of a child with Down's Syndrome, I would move heaven and earth to have the child placed under Dr. Turkel's treatment."

Dr. Allan Cott has seen similar recoveries in his large series of children he treated with orthomolecular methods, and I have seen the improvement in a few that have been referred to me.

ATTENTION DEFICIT DISORDER (ADD)

Children today suffer from a large number of serious behavioral and learning disorders which are caused primarily by the food that they eat. There is a pandemic of sick children suffering from these conditions usually called attention deficit disorder (ADD). About 20 percent of all boys entering public schools and about five percent of girls suffer from these diseases, a remarkable statistic given that in 1950 when I first started to practice psychiatry there were hardly any cases of ADD. The Kellogg Report provides an excellent description of this disorder and the factors involved. I will not repeat or summarize this report or any of the other exceptional volumes

If we do not try to improve the nutrition of our children, not only of children clearly suffering from ADD but also of almost every child in our high-tech society, we can look forward to another millennium of chronic illness, perhaps so severe as to threaten the species.

LAW

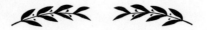

available in the alternative medical literature. Based upon this literature and on my experience with over 1,000 children I have treated I will present an outline describing the nutrition our children should be getting and the proper use of supplements. This regimen is based on my conclusion that about one third of these children have major food allergies, about one third need extra supplements, and the rest require a combination of an allergy and nutrient supplement approach. A small number will also need medication. If we do not try to improve the nutrition of our children, not only of children clearly suffering from ADD but also of almost every child in our high-tech society, we can look forward to another millennium of chronic illness, perhaps so severe as to threaten the species.

In order to treat children suffering from the poor nutrition of the modern diet, I recommend the following course of action:

1. Eliminate as much junk food as possible. The simplest way is to use the no sugar law. Processed foods usually contain a number of additives with the sugar. By eliminating this major one, most of the others are also eliminated. It is an easy rule for both the children and their parents. It is simple to advise, much more difficult to achieve.

2. Experiment with the elimination diet. The allergy history of the child and the response to foods will help to determine whether there are any food allergies. The usual allergy is towards dairy products because this is a staple food. It is more frequent in bottle fed infants. The usual history includes colic, other digestive problems, frequent colds, ear aches (often requiring tubes), rashes, itches, and later when these have subsided, hyperactivity and learning disability. There may also be a history of the child disliking milk (and being forced by mother to drink it) and loving cheese. But other foods may be involved. Often the parent will recall that after these foods the behavior of their child would

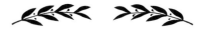

worsen in a striking manner. The child may also have a craving for that product. The final test is to place the child on a diet without these suspected foods for at least two weeks, sometimes four, and then to reintroduce them. If there was no allergy, there will be no impact on their behavior. If the child is allergic, their behavior will be better at the end of the test and will become worse when the same foods are eaten again.

When the child is very reluctant to follow any dietary changes, as many are, I will explain the value of good nutrition and invite the child to run an experiment. If they agree to follow the recommended diet very carefully for five days during the week, they can have all the junk they want on Saturdays. I tell them this is "junk" Saturday and that I want to find out if it makes them sick. They will use Sunday to get over the reaction and then on Monday will be back on the diet. Most of the children will agree to this most of the time. After they have been made ill several times, they understand the reason for the diet. Some will not and it will then require more careful persuasion from the parents to help them with the diet.

I also recommend vitamin and mineral supplements to the diet. I prefer to start with vitamin B-3 in nicotinamide form because it is less difficult for the young patient. They can tolerate the nicotinic acid flush fairly well but the flushing can annoy them, making them uncomfortable at the beginning and creating difficulty in following the program. The starting dose is 500 mg after each meal, but it may later be increased to 1 gram after each meal. It is seldom possible to go higher without running into nausea and vomiting, which must not be allowed. If the child cannot tolerate the nicotinamide, it is changed to nicotinic acid. The child and parents must be advised about the flush reaction and that it will go away in time if the vitamin is taken regularly.

If there is evidence of a vitamin B-6 dependency I add

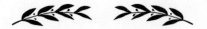

this to the program, usually 250 mg daily. It is best combined with zinc, about 15 to 30 g daily. It is particularly important for children who are autistic. Magnesium should also be given.

Every child must have enough ascorbic acid. I give them between 1.5 g and 3.0 g daily. It is a good anti-stress nutrient and decreases the frequency of colds and the flu. B-complex preparations provide extra amounts of all the B vitamins. Since it is unusual to need only one nutrient, this ensures that all these important vitamins will be provided in adequate amounts.

Perhaps 10 percent of my patients have needed a drug to help control their behavior and hyperactivity. I have found imipramine very effective, using 25 mg at night rarely going up to 75 mg. This anti-depressant is withdrawn as soon as possible. It is a good idea to take them off this drug every summer as a test, and if their behavior remains controlled when they go back to school not to restart it. With a very few schizophrenic children I have had to use major tranquilizers as well. These also are removed as soon as the child has shown an adequate response to treatment.

The child remains on this program until he is well and then for many years. It is best to keep such children on it until they are 18. However, at any time the parents may stop the program as a test, and if there is no relapse will not resume the regimen. If the child begins to relapse, they will restart the treatment.

I will give the history of only one patient to illustrate this type of response. I could write up all the cases I have seen over the past 35 years but this would be impossibly long. A case is an anecdote to the would-be scientific medical researcher but in fact medicine would not be in existence today if it were not for the use of striking cases which illustrate a point and provide direction for further research. After all, a double blind controlled experiment is only a series of anecdotes arranged in a certain way to please purists who know little about clinical medicine. They are usually

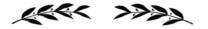

professors who see no patients, research investigators who are more interested in the Chi Sq test than in individuals, and editors and their committees who are interested only in keeping up to date with what is politically correct — and of course granting agencies who hope the Chi Sq will answer all their questions for them. I once wrote that the double blind controlled experiment is best loved by investigators with lots of money and little imagination.

One evening early in 1962, my friend Mr. A. called me at home. He was very distressed, almost in tears, as he told me about his son Ben, then nine years old. Ben had become a behavioral problem, could not learn to read, and was making so little progress in school the teaching staff had advised he be prepared for a school for slow learners or for the retarded. As he had once tested 120 on an I.Q. test, this was not only very disturbing, but extremely puzzling. I asked my friend to bring Ben to my office in the research department of the University Hospital where I was Director of Psychiatric Research so I could examine him.

Ben was a good looking, apparently healthy youngster. He denied he had any problems at school or at home. I was then inexperienced in interviewing children and could not elicit any symtomatology. As I found out later a large proportion of these children are not aware there is something wrong and tend to blame their environment for any problems which arise. Only after they are well will they recall how different they were. They develop retrospective insight for their illness.

Ben was normal at birth, sat up at 7 months, walked at 14 months, and began to speak clearly by 20 months. His parents considered him an ideal child until he was seven in Grade 2. By the end of 1960 his mother was concerned by a slight change in his behavior. He became anxious, could not fall asleep at night, or awakened frequently after he fell asleep. His mother discovered she could overcome some of the sleep difficulty by feeding him just before bed. This

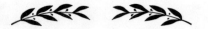

relaxed him. He continued to change, however, and school became very difficult for him. Later his parents moved to a new home and Ben was enrolled in a different school. He became more upset. This was ascribed to his difficulty in making new friends. It is a common fallacy to confuse cause and effect. Late that year his parents were shocked by his poor and erratic school performance. The teachers said he seemed to be in a shell. Reading and spelling were very poor.

In July 1961 he was referred to a mental health clinic for evaluation. He had completed Grade 3 with a D average in spite of a lot of tutoring and drilling at home by his mother, herself a teacher. When he was being taught, he seemed to understand, but soon after he could not remember what he had learned. He balked at his mother's tutoring. His mother reported that he reversed letters, had little knowledge of phonetics, and his eyes skipped back and forth or up and down so much so she used a ruler to guide his eyes on a line. He received extensive investigation from the clinic. His difficulty was ascribed to the move and/or sibling rivalry with his older brother. The clinic noted his habits of thumb sucking, nail biting, and bed wetting. They recommended remedial reading, which he received for several months with little improvement.

I ordered a mauve factor (kryptopyrrole) urine test expecting it would not show anything. To my surprise, the following morning the special area on the paper chromatogram specific for this compound was almost blood red. He was excreting large quantities of this factor. That evening I called his father and opened the conversation by saying, "George, you are in luck, Ben has schizophrenia." George wanted to know why that made him so lucky. I replied that the majority of schizophrenics excreted this factor, as did a minority of non-schizophrenic patients, and that any patient with this factor, irrespective of the diagnosis, responded to vitamin B-3 treatment. I reassured him I had not diagnosed his son schizophrenic and advised him to start Ben on nicotinamide 3 grams daily.

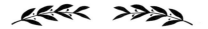

In the fall of that year George called me again. He wanted to know whether I would be interested in his son's response. He then told me that they were no longer worried because Ben was normal. Two months after he started on the vitamin the clinic giving him remedial reading discharged him as well. He had not responded to their program the previous six months. He had spent that summer happily reading books and enjoying them.

In October I received a report from a teacher who had been especially interested in him. She wrote that Mr. A. had told her Ben had not done well in school, had a reading problem, had been called stupid in school, and had therefore developed such an inferior feeling he would not answer questions. Mr. A told her that she was an expert if she could solve the case, as no other teacher had been able to.

That same afternoon the class was having dramatizations. She told them each to choose something to act out to see whether others could guess what they were doing. Each child had a turn, and to the teachers surprise, Ben too went to the front of the room to act out his part. Much to his delight he had the children guessing for quite some time, though he had acted the part very well. Later in the afternoon, after the teacher had assigned the class some work, Ben had his books out on his desk but he did not start his assignment. The teacher took Ben to the back of the room to tell her a story about some pictures she showed him. She wanted to find out the extent of his vocabulary and verbal fluency, which were remarkable. She also wanted Ben to develop a feeling of easiness with her so that he would feel free to talk to her.

The next morning the teacher left Ben more or less on his own. She did not want to push things too much. In the afternoon she taught a lesson in Social Studies. When she askcd the first question, much to her surprise, Ben raised his hand. At this moment she had to think quickly. She remembered the words of Mr. A. Ben had raised his hand. However,

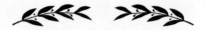

if he gave a wrong answer, others in the class might laugh at him and his inferiority would become all the more pronounced. If she did not ask him, he might never raise his hand again. The teacher took advantage of the opportunity. Ben gave the correct answer to everyone's surprise. His teacher gave him recognition and praise which he so much needed. From then on Ben continued to volunteer answers in group discussions and took an active interest in classroom activities.

This teacher reported many improvements, physically, socially, emotionally, and educationally. At the beginning of the term, Ben took pride in the fact that his mother was a teacher. Later on in the term, Ben also started to mention his father and brother. Ben was no longer shy. He became a sparkling personality, not afraid to speak up. He started to take an interest in sports, in which he excelled. He got along well with the children at school and at camp. He assumed leadership and organization duties. He read with eye-reversal not noticeable in reading and seldom in writing. Ben went on the stage to sing, make a speech, and read the morning scripture to the whole student body and the staff. All of these things he did well with little noticeable nervousness and tension.

Early in 1966 his father told me Ben had made A's and B's in Grade 7. In May 1968 he participated in a track meet, was active in extra curricular activities, had been a stage manager for a high school play. His parents considered him to be normal. I examined him for the last time in August 1970. He was well. Since then Ben has remained normal. He is an outdoors professional, fully employed in a permanent position, and happily married with two children.

ORTHOMOLECULAR
HEALTH-CARE

ECONOMICAL

The direct costs of treating disease are the costs of the physicians services; the cost of other health care services such as nursing, social work, physiotherapy, and psychological services; and the costs of drugs and nutrients. The cost of physicians services is usually calculated either on a fee for service basis or by annual salaries. With physicians on annual salary, one seldom divides the number of patients into their salary to determine what the costs are. The fee for each visit or each procedure does not give an accurate estimate of the total cost of treatment. For example, a physician may see a patient 100 times over a two year period, while another physician might be a better diagnostician and treat that patient successfully in 10 visits. The more accurate cost is the cost of getting each patient well. A doctor charging $10,000 to cure a patient may be providing a very economical service compared to a physician who sees the patient for five years and charges $25,000 dollars. The fee is a valid measure of costs only if every doctor were equally skillful, equally dedicated, and used similar treatment methods.

Orthomolecular treatment is much more economical for two reasons. The most important is that it leads to recoveries in a shorter period of time and requires fewer visits to the

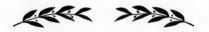

doctor. This is why orthomolecular psychiatrists can see many more patients than do psychiatrists who place more faith in psychotherapy or drugs. There is nothing more economical than to get the patient normal quickly. Secondly, orthomolecular medicine reduces the costs of drugs. Each year for the past 25 years I have examined my pattern of practice (a profile provided by the medicare program) and compared it against the average of all the psychiatrists practicing in Saskatchewan and since 1976 in British Columbia. Each year I have seen nearly twice as many patients compared to the mean for all the psychiatrists, and my billings to the governments have been about 10 percent higher than for the average billing. I do not work particularly hard, and for the past 10 years have been seeing patients only four days each week. If every psychiatrist practiced the way I do, we would need 50 percent fewer psychiatrists for the same population in North America.

The best way to compare costs is to examine several case histories of patients which are representative of a few diseases.

Arthritis

Dr. W. Kaufman showed that nicotinamide in doses up to 4 grams daily was therapeutic for arthritis. He was a very careful clinician and used the best clinical methods, including devices he had made for measuring the degree of joint movement and function. But his work remained totally invisible to the medical establishment for several reasons.

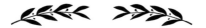

Vitamins were then *known* not to be therapeutic for anything except to prevent deficiency diseases such as pellagra. About that time the wonder drugs, corticosteroids and ACTH, exploded on the world medical scene with a Nobel Prize awarded to one of the Mayo Clinic scientists who developed the drugs and a patent was granted to Merck and Co. Since then the attention of all rheumatologists has centered on the use of corticosteroids, even though they have limited usefulness. A double blind experiment in England around 1949 showed that aspirin was as effective as the steroids, but this did not dampen much the enthusiasm for these drugs. I have seen how effective vitamin B-3 is for the treatment of arthritis. The early cases respond rapidly, the chronic cases more slowly. The saving in time and drug costs is enormous, as is the rapidity of the response for early cases who do not go on to become chronic as they do with drugs.

Crohns Disease

I have treated many cases of Crohns disease in the past 20 years. The basic treatment is to eliminate dairy products, eliminate wheat and perhaps all the grasses, and to use vitamins and minerals. The B-vitamins are very important, as is vitamin E which is used in doses up to 4000 i.u. daily. I think Crohns disease is an example of a double deficiency or double dependency disease. My most recent example is a young woman who had a very severe form with a lot of bleeding. The year before I saw her she had been in hospital at least four times requiring transfusions of blood each time. Her hospital record was at at least two inches thick. She was placed on the program, and for the past four months has been well. She is still on very small doses of steroids, compared to the much larger doses she had needed before. The saving in hospital costs and medical costs will be substantial. She is not the only case. In the past year I have seen three more patients who are responding as well.

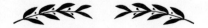

Heart Disease

The two most common heart conditions are hypercholesterolemia and hypertension. Cardiovascular disease is a major cause of death and disability. Standard treatment includes modification of the diet by decreasing the fat intake and the use of drugs for lowering cholesterol levels when the diet alone will not do so. The shift in diet is desirable and not expensive since it calls for a decrease in the consumption of the more expensive foods, such as dairy products and meats. The drugs for lowering cholesterol are very expensive, running around $100 per month or more. And they have not been shown to decrease overall mortality and morbidity.

Orthomolecular therapy also seeks to change the diet by lowering total fat intake and also by eliminating the sugars. The diet to which we had adapted automatically lowers fat appreciably and eliminates the simple sugars. If these simple dietary measures do not work, one can add nicotinic acid, which is an effective substance for lowering cholesterol and elevating HDL and which has been shown to decrease mortality and morbidity. This has been discussed under vitamin B-3. A combined supplement regimen, including ample vitamin C, vitamin B-6, nicotinic acid, and folic acid, will ensure that these cardiovascular problems will not develop if the program is started well before permanent damage has been done. Nicotinic acid alone taken over 18 months has removed a lot of plaque from blood vessels and increased the diameter. Nicotinic acid will cost around $10 per month but the improved none-flush linodil ester will cost three times as much.

Hypertension can be treated by making sure the ratio of potassium over sodium is high, perhaps three to one. The diet to which we had adapted will provide this ratio. Most of the sodium in our diet is derived from processed foods which are salted in order to replace an agreeable taste with the flatter taste of the processed food from which the natural flavor and taste have been removed. This diet will be compatible

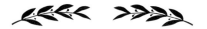

with any drug treatment necessary to reduce elevated pressure. In many cases, this diet plus the use of supplements has allowed a gradual withdrawal from anti-hypertensive drugs.

Peptic Ulcer

Many patients with peptic ulcer are allergic to a food or several foods. A common allergy is to dairy products, but when I studied medicine the common treatment for peptic ulcer was the Sippi diet, a high milk, frequent feeding diet. The hypothesis was that the milk would absorb all that excess hydrochloric acid and thus allow the ulcer to heal. Today, few physicians still use the Sippi diets. I have seen several patients whose ulcer improved and vanished when they were placed on a diet which eliminated what they were allergic to. This would be much cheaper for them than to have to take very expensive drugs required to control excess secretion of acid. These drugs are very helpful and might be needed even with such a diet, but the likelihood they will be required for long periods of time is greatly diminished with the proper diet and the use of supplements.

Psychiatric Diseases

The differences in the cost of treatment between traditional and alternative orthomolecular medicine are much clearer when psychiatric patients are treated, for the difference is between patients who remain chronic and require care and treatment the rest of their lives and patients who recover and take charge of their own lives. Standard psychiatric treatment may be psychotherapy alone or combined with medication, or it may consist only of medication with psychiatric support and supervision of the medication. Psychotherapy alone requires many treatment sessions and may continue for many months and often for many years at weekly or monthly intervals. This is not a criticism, for if the therapy is successful it is worth it. However, psychotherapy alone is singularly ineffective. There are several hundred

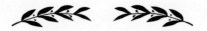

studies showing how the results of psychotherapy are no better than chance and hardly any studies showing that it can
do better than simply leaving the patient alone. The antidepressants are much more effective for the various kinds of
depression. Tranquilizers are helpful in treating schizophrenics but do not enable the patient to recover. On the
contrary, patients on tranquilizers will not recover to the
point that they can become independent members of society. With orthomolecular psychiatry, a much greater proportion of the patients recover to the point that they pay income
tax. Every schizophrenic teenager will over their lifetime cost
the state or province over two million dollars. This will be
the accumulated cost of hospital treatment, welfare, medical
costs, drug costs, and cost of lost income, for they will hardly
ever be able to work again at jobs remotely like the one they
had before they became sick. Other costs include legal and
police costs. The loss due to the destruction of the patient
and often of their family cannot be calculated. Here are a
few examples.

A woman had been depressed for twenty years. She had
not responded to medication, to psychiatric treatment, or to
a stay in a mental hospital where she was given ECT. She saw
me on a Friday and I determined she probably suffered from
a dairy allergy. I advised her to discontinue all dairy products. The following Monday she was free of depression. This
rapid response is rare, but a large number of depressions
have shown equally striking recoveries, although it has taken
them at least two weeks to achieve. The use of diet and supplements has greatly decreased the need for large doses of
anti-depressant. I routinely use half the usual recommended
dose when I prescribe them at all.

In 1960 a doctor from California called me. He was
very depressed and cried as he told me about his son, then
twelve years old, who was in a university psychiatric hospital
in Palo Alto. He had just been advised by his son's psychiatrist that he would never recover and that the only thing

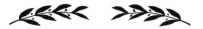

left for him would be to transfer him to a mental hospital. After that frightening advice, he began to read as much as he could in the medical library and discovered the first paper we had published in 1957 where we described the use of vitamin B-3 for the treatment of schizophrenia.

I recommended he obtain nicotinic acid and give his son 1 gram three times each day. In 1960 no company was making these large sized doses. The smaller 100 mg tablets were useless because they contained so much filler that the correct dose, 30 tablets daily, would make them sick from the fillers. The physician contacted a drug company who agreed to make the 500 mg tablets for him. When his supply arrived, he took it to the hospital and asked the psychiatrist to start his son on it. The psychiatrist became very angry and promptly came back with two lies. He told the father that they had tried the vitamin and that it had not done any good, then added that it would fry his brain. He concluded by warning the father that if he insisted his son would be discharged. He was too psychotic to be discharged.

The father then decided he was going to have his son take the vitamin without the psychiatrist's knowledge. He ground up each tablet and placed one gram on a slice of bread. This he covered with jam. Each day he appeared at the hospital to visit his son and to feed him jam sandwiches. After a few weeks he became worried that the psychiatrist might find out because his son said to him, "Daddy, whenever I eat that sandwich I turn red." He promptly changed the nicotinic acid to nicotinamide. After twelve weeks the boy said he wanted to go home. He was discharged and completed high school in the top 95 percentile for the United States. He went to university, took medicine, graduated, and is now a research psychiatrist. Had he not been on this vitamin the state would have faced enormous costs, as would his family, and he would be a chronic patient today. Instead he is a normal productive psychiatrist doing research and paying income tax.

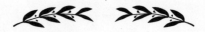

How does one compare these two kinds of results. It is very simple. The vast majority of schizophrenics never do recover. The vast proportion of early schizophrenic patients do when they are treated by orthomolecular methods. I know personally 17 men and women practicing medicine and psychiatry who were all teen-age schizophrenics. On the orthomolecular regimen they have recovered. Several have academic appointments. One was the president of a major psychiatric association for one year.

Here are a couple of brief case histories out of about 1500 children under age 14 I have seen since 1955. The first one I did not treat. Several years ago a mother brought her seven-year-old son to me. On examination he appeared normal. She then told me that he had been diagnosed autistic by a clinic in Victoria. He had been given the best possible treatment, but there had been no response. She had read about the connection between allergies and abnormal behavior. She thought her son might be allergic to milk. She discussed it with the health professionals at the clinic, who laughed at her and made her feel very foolish. However, this did not deter her, and on her own she placed him on a dairy free and sugar free diet. One month later he was normal. She then took him back to the clinic. They apologized to her for their previous attitude. Still, she wanted some medical sanction that she was doing the right thing and came to me for this.

The second case was a young boy in public school. He was hyperactive and had a learning disorder. Out of 20 in his class he was at the bottom. I took him off dairy products and sugar and started him on nicotinamide 1 gram, three times per day, with the same amount of vitamin C and 250 mg of vitamin B-6. By spring he was at the head of his class. How would one estimate the costs to the boy, his family, and society if he had not been treated and was left permanently impaired by no education and a total inability to take his normal place in society?

To lower costs, the medical profession will need to adopt

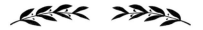

the principles and practices of orthomolecular or nutritional medicine and psychiatry. This will be achieved two main ways. (1) Increase the amount of information on the value of good nutrition and nutrient supplements for the public and for the profession. The public is already getting more and more information since the major media have lost their fear of so-called alternative health practices and the profession is also beginning to get more in the form of reports, articles in the medical journals, and papers delivered at medical meetings. (2) Make it possible for physicians to practice nutritional medicine. The medical establishment must remove the fear that physicians will lose their medical license if they begin to work with vitamins and minerals.

> *To lower costs, the medical profession will need to adopt the principles and practices of orthomolecular or nutritional medicine and psychiatry.*

LAW

RESPONSIBLE

The pressure on physicians to conform has been immense and many physicians have lost their license because they would not give up their practice of nutritional medicine. The pressure is lessening but is still present. I know many doctors who would be very interested in practicing this way but are afraid they will lose their livelihood. The worst offenders are the official bodies, such as the Colleges of Physician and Surgeons in Canada. In the Province of British Columbia, they are trying to suppress the use of chelation therapy, considering it dangerous and not proven. They are wrong on both counts but accuracy seems of little interest to them. I suspect the suppression of chelation therapy will be reversed only when governments force the regulatory bodies to cease their opposition.

In 1990, a legislative bill was passed in Washington State stating that the medical board may not base a finding of professional incompetence solely on the basis that a licensee's practice is unconventional or experimental in the absence of demonstrable physical harm to the patient. In 1992 Alaska Governor Walter J. Hickel appointed Dr. R. Rowento to the medical board, who stated, against the protests of many fellow physicians, that "there is as much room for divergent opinions in medicine as there are for divergent beliefs in God. I have stated it is time for medicine to be responsible to the people rather than to the needs of the profession. Organized medicine must take an honest look at itself, acknowledge that it does not have all the answers and reach out to embrace other avenues to healing as both orthodox and complementary medicine have much to offer. Each can fill in some of the gaps left by the other." I could not have stated my own position better. Embracing this belief in the value of nutritional health care, we can look forward to a new age of good health for all in the twenty-first century.

> **LAW**
>
> *Embracing this belief in the value of nutritional health care, we can look forward to a new age of good health for all in the twenty-first century.*

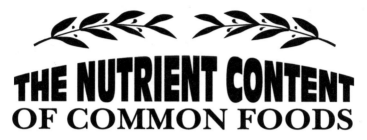

THE NUTRIENT CONTENT
OF COMMON FOODS

THE NUTRIENT CONTENT
OF COMMON FOODS

❦

I t is always best to acquire all of the daily allotment of nutrients you need from the nutritional quality of foods eaten.
The following list of the vitamin and mineral content of many
foods will help you tailor your eating to your specific dietary
needs. Use the listing to identify foods that are good sources
for the particular vitamin or mineral you are interested in.

While the values given in these lists can be useful in comparing nutritional content in foods, the absolute values for
food nutrients will vary, depending on such factors as the
condition of the soil where the food was grown (or what type
of nutrition an animal received), the amount of processing
or refining, and the method of preparation.

LAW
*It is always best to acquire all of the daily allotment of nutrients
you need from the nutritional quality of foods eaten.*

The serving size of each food in the lists has been stan-
dardized to 100 grams. This was done to provide a more
appropriate comparison between the relative amounts of
nutrients in foods and allows them to be ranked from highest to lowest. Remember, however, not all foods are consumed
in 100-gram quantities, especially if they are highly concentrated, like kelp, dulse, wheat germ, and brewer's yeast. Such
foods often appear at the top of the list, indicating that they
are concentrated nutritional sources. To get an idea of what

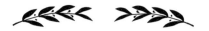

100 grams of a food represents, it may be helpful to consider what it is equivalent to in common measurements. A 100-gram serving size is approximately equal to any one of the following:

- about 3/8 cup fluid measure
- about 1/4 cup dry measure
- 3 1/4 ounces of milk or yogurt
- slightly more than 1 cup leafy vegetable
- 3/4 cup root vegetable
- 5 1/2 ounces nuts, seeds
- 2/3 cup of sliced fruit
- 1/2 cup cereal grain, uncooked
- 7 tablespoons cooking oil
- 5 tablespoons honey, molasses

The following lists indicate the amounts of important nutrients available in 100-gram portions of various foods.

VITAMINS

VITAMIN A (*Carotene*)

I.U. per 100-gram (3 1/2 oz) portion		I.U. per 100-gram (3 1/2 oz) portion	
50,500	Lamb liver	43,900	Beef liver
22,500	Calf liver	21,600	Peppers, red chili
14,000	Dandelion greens	12,100	Chicken liver
11,000	Carrots	10,900	Apricots,dried
9,300	Collard leaves	8,900	Kale
8,800	Sweet potatoes	8,500	Parsley
8,100	Spinach	7,600	Turnip greens
7,000	Mustard greens	6,500	Swiss chard
6,100	Beet greens	5,800	Chives
5,700	Butternut squash	4,900	Watercress
4,800	Mangos	4,450	Peppers, sweet red
4,300	Hubbard squash	3,400	Cantaloupe

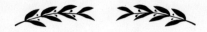

3,300	Endive	2,700	Apricots
2,500	Broccoli spears	2,260	Whitefish
2,000	Green onions	1,900	Romaine lettuce
1,750	Papayas	1,650	Nectarines
1,600	Prunes	1,600	Pumpkin
1,580	Swordfish	1,540	Whipping cream
1,330	Peaches	1,200	Acorn squash
1,180	Eggs	1,080	Chicken
1,000	Cherries, sour red	970	Butterhead lettuce
900	Asparagus	900	Tomatoes, ripe
770	Peppers, green chili	690	Kidneys
640	Peas	600	Green beans
600	Elderberries	590	Watermelon
580	Rutabagas	550	Brussels sprouts
520	Okra	510	Yellow cornmeal
460	Yellow squash		

Vitamin A from animal source foods occurs mostly as active, pre-formed vitamin A (retinol), while that from vegetable source foods occurs as pro-vitamin A (beta-carotene and other carotenoids) that must be converted to active vitamin A by the body to be utilized. The efficiency of conversion varies among individuals; however, beta-carotene is converted more efficiently than other carotenoids. Green and deep-yellow vegetables, as well as deep-yellow fruits, are highest in beta-carotene.

VITAMIN B1 (*Thiamin*)

I.U. per 100-gram (3^1/$_2$ oz) portion		I.U. per 100-gram (3^1/$_2$ oz) portion	
15.61	Brewer's yeast	14.01	Torula yeast
2.01	Wheat germ	1.96	Sunflower seeds
1.84	Rice polishings	1.28	Pine nuts
1.14	Peanuts, with skins	1.10	Soybeans, dry
1.05	Cowpeas, dry	.98	Peanuts, without skins
.96	Brazil nuts	.93	Pork, lean
.86	Pecans	.85	Soybean flour

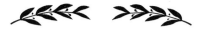

.84	Beans, pinto and red	.74	Split peas
.73	Millet	.72	Wheat bran
.67	Pistachio nuts	.65	Navy beans
.63	Veal, heart	.60	Buckwheat
.60	Oatmeal	.55	Whole wheat flour
.55	Whole wheat	.51	Lamb kidneys
.31	Garbanzos	.48	Lima beans, dry
.46	Hazelnuts	.45	Lamb heart
.45	Wild rice	.43	Cashews
.43	Rye, whole grain	.40	Lamb liver
.40	Lobster	.38	Mung beans
.38	Cornmeal, whole	.37	Lentils
.36	Beef kidneys	.35	Green peas
.34	Brown rice	.33	Walnuts
.30	Pork liver	.25	Garlic, cloves
.25	Beef Liver	.24	Almonds ground
.24	Lima beans, fresh	.24	Pumpkin and squash seeds
.23	Brains, all kinds	.23	Soybean sprouts
.22	Peppers, red chili		

VITAMIN B2 (*Riboflavin*)

I.U. per 100-gram (3½ oz) portion		I.U. per 100-gram (3½ oz) portion	
5.06	Torula yeast	4.28	Brewer's yeast
3.28	Lamb liver	3.26	Beef liver
3.03	Pork liver	2.72	Calf liver
2.55	Beef kidneys	2.49	Chicken liver
2.42	Lamb kidneys	1.36	Chicken giblets
1.05	Veal heart	.92	Almonds
.88	Beef heart	.74	Lamb heart
.68	Wheat germ	.63	Wild rice
.46	Mushrooms	.44	Egg yolks
.38	Millet	.36	Peppers, hot red
.35	Soy flour	.35	Wheat bran
.33	Mackerel	.31	Collards
.31	Soybeans, dry	.30	Eggs

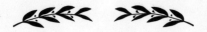

.29	Split peas	.29	Beef tongue
.29	Brains, all kinds	.26	Kale
.26	Parsley	.25	Cashews
.25	Rice bran	.25	Veal
.24	Lamb, lean	.23	Broccoli
.23	Chicken, meat and skin	.23	Pine nuts
.23	Salmon	.23	Sunflower seeds .
.22	Rye, whole grain	.22	Navy beans
.22	Beet and Mustard greens	.21	Beans, pinto and red
.22	Lentils	.22	Pork, lean
.22	Prunes	.21	Mung beans
.21	Blackeyed peas	.21	Okra
.13	Sesame seeds, hulled		

VITAMIN B3 (*Niacin*)

I.U. per 100-gram (3½ oz) portion		I.U. per 100-gram (3½ oz) portion	
44.4	Torula yeast	37.9	Brewer's yeast
29.8	Rice bran	28.2	Rice polishings
21.0	Wheat bran	17.2	Peanuts, with skins
16.9	Lamb liver	16.4	Pork liver
15.8	Peanuts, without skins	13.6	Beef liver
11.4	Calf liver	11.3	Turkey, light meat
10.8	Chicken liver	10.7	Chicken, light meat
8.4	Trout	8.3	Halibut
8.2	Mackerel	8.1	Veal heart
8.0	Chicken, meat only	8.0	Swordfish
8.0	Turkey, meat only	7.7	Goose, meat only
7.5	Beef heart	7.2	Salmon
6.4	Veal	6.4	Beef kidneys
6.2	Wild rice	6.1	Chicken giblets
5.7	Lamb, lean	5.6	Chicken, meat & skin
5.4	Sesame seeds	5.4	Sunflower seeds
5.1	Beef, lean	5.0	Pork, lean
4.7	Brown rice	4.5	Pine nuts
4.4	Buckwheat, whole grain	4.4	Peppers, red chili

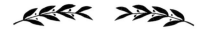

4.4	Whole wheat grain	4.3	Whole whet flour
4.2	Mushrooms	4.2	Wheat germ
3.7	Barley	3.6	Herring
3.5	Almonds	3.5	Shrimp
3.0	Haddock	3.0	Split peas

PANTOTHENIC ACID (*a B vitamin*)

I.U. per 100-gram (3½ oz) portion		I.U. per 100-gram (3½ oz) portion	
12.0	Brewer's yeast	11.0	Torula yeast
8.0	Calf liver	6.0	Chicken liver
3.9	Beef kidneys	2.8	Peanuts
2.6	Brains, all kinds	2.6	Heart
2.2	Mushrooms	2.0	Soybean flour
2.0	Split peas	2.0	Beef tongue
1.9	Perch	1.8	Blue cheese
1.7	Pecans	1.7	Soybeans
1.6	Eggs	1.5	Lobster
1.5	Oatmeal, dry	1.4	Buckwheat flour
1.4	Sunflower seeds	1.4	Lentils
1.3	Rye flour, whole	1.3	Cashews
1.3	Salmon	1.2	Camembert cheese
1.2	Garbanzos	1.2	Wheat germ, toasted
1.2	Broccoli	1.1	Hazelnuts
1.1	Turkey, dark meat	1.1	Brown rice
1.1	Wheat flour, whole	1.1	Sardines
1.1	Peppers, red chili	1.1	Avocados
1.1	Veal, lean	1.0	Blackeyed peas, dry
1.0	Wild rice	1.0	Cauliflower
1.0	Chicken, dark meat	1.0	Kale

VITAMIN B6 (*Pyridoxine*)

I.U. per 100-gram (3½ oz) portion		I.U. per 100-gram (3½ oz) portion	
3.00	Torula yeast	2.50	Brewer's yeast

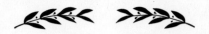

1.25	Sunflower seeds	1.15	Wheat germ, toasted
.90	Tuna	.84	Beef liver
.81	Soybeans, dry	.75	Chicken liver
.73	Walnuts	.70	Salmon
.69	Trout	.67	Calf liver
.66	Mackerel	.65	Pork liver
.63	Soybean flour	.60	Lentils, dry
.58	Buckwheat flour	.58	Lima beans, dry
.56	Blackeyed peas, dry	.56	Navy beans, dry
.55	Brown rice	.54	Garbanzos, dry
.53	Pinto beans, dry	.51	Bananas
.45	Pork, lean	.44	Albacore
.43	Beef, lean	.43	Halibut
.43	Beef kidneys	.42	Avocados
.41	Veal kidneys	.34	Whole wheat flour
.33	Chestnuts, fresh	.30	Egg yolks
.30	Kale	.30	Rye flour
.28	Spinach	.26	Turnip greens
.25	Beef heart	.26	Peppers, sweet
.25	Potatoes	.24	Prunes
.24	Raisins	.24	Sardines
.24	Brussels Sprouts	.23	Elderberries
.23	Perch	.22	Cod
.22	Barley	.22	Camembert cheese
.22	Sweet potatoes	.21	Cauliflower
.20	Popcorn, popped	.20	Red cabbage
.20	Leeks	.20	Molasses

FOLIC ACID (*a B vitamin*)

I.U. per 100-gram (3½ oz) portion		I.U. per 100-gram (3½ oz) portion	
2022	Brewer's yeast	440	Blackeyed peas
430	Rice germ	425	Soy flour
305	Wheat germ	295	Beef liver
275	Lamb liver	225	Soybeans
220	Pork liver	195	Bran

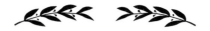

180	Kidney beans	145	Mung beans
130	Lima beans	125	Navy beans
125	Garbanzos	110	Asparagus
105	Lentils	77	Walnuts
75	Spinach, fresh	70	Kale
65	Filbert nuts	60	Beet and Mustard greens
57	Textured vegetable protein	56	Peanuts, roasted
		56	Peanut butter
53	Broccoli	50	Barley
50	Split peas	49	Whole wheat cereal
49	Brussels sprouts	45	Almonds
38	Whole wheat flour	33	Oatmeal
32	Dried figs	30	Avocado
28	Green beans	28	Corn
28	Coconut, fresh	27	Pecans
25	Mushrooms	25	Dates
14	Blackberries	7	Ground beef
5	Oranges		

VITAMIN B12 (*Cobalamin*)

I.U. per 100-gram (3 1/2 oz) portion		I.U. per 100-gram (3 1/2 oz) portion	
104	Lamb liver	98	Clams
80	Beef liver	63	Lamb kidneys
60	Calf liver	31	Beef kidneys
25	Chicken liver	18	Oysters
17	Sardines	11	Beef heart
6	Egg yolks	5.2	Lamb heart
5.0	Trout	4.0	Brains, all kinds
4.0	Salmon	3.0	Tuna
2.1	Lamb	2.1	Sweetbreads
2.0	Eggs	2.0	Whey, dried
1.8	Beef, lean	1.8	Edam cheese
1.8	Swiss cheese	1.6	Brie cheese
1.6	Gruyere cheese	1.4	Blue cheese
1.3	Haddock	1.2	Flounder

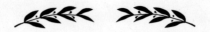

1.2	Scallops	1.0	Cheddar cheese
1.0	Cottage cheese	1.0	Mozzarella cheese
1.0	Halibut	1.0	Perch, fillets
1.0	Swordfish		

BIOTIN (*a B vitamin*)

I.U. per 100-gram (3½ oz) portion		I.U. per 100-gram (3½ oz) portion	
200	Brewer's Yeast	127	Lamb liver
100	Pork liver	96	Beef liver
70	Soy flour	61	Soybeans
60	Rice bran	58	Rice germ
57	Rice polishings	52	Egg yolk
39	Peanut butter	37	Walnuts
34	Peanuts, roasted	31	Barley
27	Pecans	24	Oatmeal
24	Sardines, canned	22	Eggs
21	Blackeyed peas	18	Split peas
18	Almonds	17	Cauliflower
16	Mushrooms	16	Whole wheat cereal
15	Salmon, canned	15	Textured vegetable protein
14	Bran	13	Lentils
12	Brown rice	10	Chicken

CHOLINE (*a B vitamin*)

I.U. per 100-gram (3½ oz) portion		I.U. per 100-gram (3½ oz) portion	
2200	Lecithin	1490	Egg yolk
550	Liver	504	Whole eggs
406	Wheat germ	340	Soybeans
300	Rice germ	257	Blackeyed peas
245	Garbanzo beans	240	Brewer's yeast
223	Lentils	201	Split peas
170	Rice bran	162	Peanuts, roasted

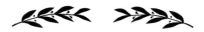

156	Oatmeal	145	Peanut butter
143	Bran	139	Barley
122	Ham	112	Brown rice
104	Veal	102	Rice polishings
94	Whole wheat cereal	86	Molasses
77	Pork	75	Beef
75	Green peas	48	Cheddar cheese
66	Sweet potatoes	42	Green beans
29	Potatoes	23	Cabbage
22	Spinach	20.5	Textured vegetable protein
15	Milk	12	Orange juice
5	Butter		

INOSITOL (*a B vitamin*)

I.U. per
100-gram (3½ oz) portion

I.U. per
100-gram (3½ oz) portion

2220	Lecithin	770	Wheat germ
500	Navy beans	460	Rice bran
454	Rice polishings	390	Barley, cooked
370	Rice germ	370	Whole Wheat
270	Brewer's yeast	270	Oatmeal
240	Blackeyed peas	240	Garbanzo beans
210	Oranges	205	Soy flour
200	Soybeans	180	Peanuts, roasted
180	Peanut butter	170	Lima beans
162	Green peas	150	Molasses
150	Grapefruit	150	Split peas
130	Lentils	120	Raisins
120	Cantaloupe	119	Brown rice
117	Orange juice	110	Whole wheat flour
96	Peaches	95	Cabbage
95	Cauliflower	88	Onions
67	Whole wheat bread	66	Sweet potatoes
64	Watermelon	60	Strawberries
55	Lettuce	51	Beef liver

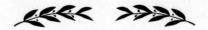

46	Tomatoes	33	Eggs
13	Milk	11	Beef, round

VITAMIN B17 (*Amygdalin*)

For certain nutrients, there are few foods sources that contain appreciable quantities. In these cases we list those foods that are best sources, rather than relative nutrient amounts.

Foods containing more than 500 milligrams per 100-gram portion:

Wild blackberries	Apple seeds	Cherry seeds
Elderberries	Apricot seeds	Nectarine seeds
Peach seeds	Fava beans	Bamboo sprouts
Pear seeds	Mung beans	Alfalfa leaves
Plum seeds	Bitter almonds	
Prune seeds	Macadamia nuts	

Foods containing between 100 and 500 milligrams per 100-gram portion:

Boysenberries	Raspberries	Garbanzo beans
Currants	Alfalfa sprouts	Blackeyed peas
Gooseberries	Buckwheat	Kidney beans
Huckleberries	Flax seed	Lentils
Loganberries	Millet	Lima beans
Mulberries	Squash seed	
Quince	Mung bean sprouts	

Foods containing below 100 milligrams per 100-gram portion:

Commercial blackberries	Peas	Cashews
Cranberries	Lima beans	Beet tops
Black beans	Sweet potatoes, yams	

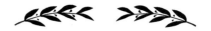

PARA-AMINOBENZOIC ACID (PABA)
(*a B vitamin*)

Good sources include:

Mushrooms	Sunflower seeds	Whole milk
Liver	Wheat germ	Eggs
Bran	Oats	
Cabbage	Spinach	

PANGAMIC ACID (*Vitamin B15*)

Good sources include:

Apricot kernels	Corn grits	Oat grits
Yeast	Wheat germ	Sunflower seeds
Liver	Wheat bran	Pumpkin seeds
Rice bran		

VITAMIN C (*Ascorbic Acid*)

I.U. per 100-gram (3½ oz) portion		I.U. per 100-gram (3½ oz) portion	
1300	Acerola	369	Peppers, red chili
242	Guavas	204	Peppers, red sweet
186	Kale leaves	172	Parsley
152	Collard leaves	139	Turnip greens
128	Peppers, green sweet	113	Broccoli
102	Brussels sprouts	97	Mustard greens
79	Watercress	78	Cauliflower
66	Persimmons	61	Cabbage, red
59	Strawberries	56	Papayas
51	Spinach	50	Oranges and juice
47	Cabbage	46	Lemon juice
38	Grapefruit and juice	36	Elderberries
36	Calf liver	36	Turnips

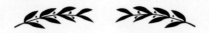

35	Mangoes	33	Asparagus
33	Cantaloupes	32	Swiss chard
32	Green onions	31	Beef liver
31	Okra	31	Tangerines
30	New Zealand spinach	30	Oysters
29	Lima beans, young	29	Blackeyed beans
29	Soybeans	27	Green peas
26	Radishes	25	Raspberries
25	Chinese cabbage	25	Yellow summer squash
24	Loganberries	23	Honeydew melon
23	Tomatoes	23	Pork liver

VITAMIN D

I.U. per		I.U. per	
100-gram (3½ oz) portion		100-gram (3½ oz) portion	
500	Sardines, canned	350	Salmon
250	Tuna	150	Shrimp
90	Sunflower seeds	90	Butter
50	Liver	50	Eggs
40	Milk, fortified	40	Mushrooms
30	Natural cheeses		

VITAMIN E (*Tocopherol*)

I.U. per		I.U. per	
100-gram (3½ oz) portion		100-gram (3½ oz) portion	
216	Wheat germ oil	90	Sunflower seeds
88	Sunflower seed oil	72	Safflower oil
48	Almonds	45	Sesame oil
34	Peanut oil	29	Corn oil
22	Wheat germ	18	Olive oil
18	Peanuts	14	Soybean oil
13	Peanuts, roasted	11	Peanut butter
3.0	Bran	3.6	Butter
3.2	Spinach	3.0	Oatmeal

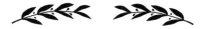

2.9	Asparagus		2.5	Salmon
2.5	Brown rice		2.3	Rye, whole
2.2	Rye bread, dark		1.9	Pecans
1.9	Wheat germ		1.9	Rye and wheat crackers
1.4	Whole wheat bread		1.0	Carrots
0.99	Peas		0.92	Walnuts
0.88	Bananas		0.83	Eggs
0.72	Tomatoes		0.29	Lamb

VITAMIN K

I.U. per 100-gram (3½ oz) portion		I.U. per 100-gram (3½ oz) portion	
650	Turnip greens	200	Broccoli
129	Lettuce	125	Cabbage
92	Beef liver	89	Spinach
57	Watercress	57	Asparagus
35	Cheese	30	Butter
25	Pork liver	20	Oats
19	Green peas	17	Whole wheat
14	Green beans	11	Pork
11	Eggs	10	Corn oil
8	Peaches	7	Beef
7	Chicken liver	6	Raisins
5	Tomatoes	3	Milk
3	Potatoes		

BIOFLAVONOIDS (*Vitamin P*)

Goods sources include:

Grapes	Black currants	Peppers
Rose hips	Plums	Papaya
Prunes	Parsley	Cantaloupe
Oranges	Grapefruit	Tomatoes
Lemon juice	Cabbage	Cherries
Apricots		

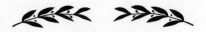

MINERALS

CALCIUM

I.U. per 100-gram (3½ oz) portion		I.U. per 100-gram (3½ oz) portion	
1093	Kelp	925	Swiss cheese
750	Cheddar cheese	352	Carob flour
296	Dulse	250	Collard leaves
246	Turnip greens	245	Barbados molasses
234	Almonds	210	Brewer's yeast
203	Parsley	200	Corn tortillas (lime added)
187	Dandelion greens	186	Brazil nuts
151	Watercress	129	Goat's milk
128	Tofu	126	Dried figs
121	Buttermilk	120	Sunflower seeds
120	Yogurt	119	Beet greens
119	Wheat bran	118	Whole milk
114	Buckwheat, raw	110	Sesame seeds, hulled
106	Ripe olives	103	Broccoli
99	English walnut	94	Cottage cheese
93	Spinach	73	Soybeans, cooked
73	Pecans	72	Wheat germ
69	Peanuts	68	Miso
68	Romaine lettuce	67	Dried apricots
66	Rutabaga	62	Raisins
60	Black currants	59	Dates
56	Green snap beans	51	Globe artichokes
51	Dried prunes	51	Pumpkin and squash seeds
50	Cooked dry beans		
49	Common cabbage	48	Soybean sprouts
46	Hard winter wheat	41	Oranges
39	Celery	38	Cashews
38	Rye grain	37	Carrots
34	Barley	32	Sweet potatoes
32	Brown rice	29	Garlic
28	Summer squash	27	Onions

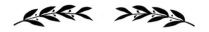

26	Lemons	26	Fresh green peas
25	Cauliflower	25	Lentils, cooked
22	Sweet cherries	22	Asparagus
22	Winter squash	21	Strawberry
20	Millet	19	Mung bean sprouts
17	Pineapple	16	Grapes
16	Beets	14	Cantaloupe
14	Jerusalem artichokes	13	Tomatoes
12	Eggplant	12	Chicken
11	Orange juice	10	Avocado
10	Beef	8	Bananas
7	Apples	3	Sweet corn

MAGNESIUM

I.U. per		I.U. per	
100-gram (3½ oz) portion		100-gram (3½ oz) portion	
760	Kelp	490	Wheat bran
336	Wheat germ	270	Almonds
267	Cashews	258	Blackstrap molasses
231	Brewer's yeast	229	Buckwheat
225	Brazil nuts	220	Dulse
184	Filberts	175	Peanuts
162	Millet	160	Wheat grain
142	Pecan	131	English walnut
115	Rye	111	Tofu
106	Beet greens	90	Coconut meat, dry
88	Soybeans, cooked	88	Spinach
88	Brown rice	71	Dried figs
65	Swiss chard	62	Apricots, dried
58	Dates	57	Collard leaves
51	Shrimp	48	Sweet corn
45	Cheddar cheese	41	Parsley
40	Prunes, dried	38	Sunflower seeds
37	Common beans, cooked	37	Barley
36	Dandelion greens	36	Garlic
36	Raisins	35	Fresh green peas

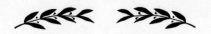

34	Potatoes with skin	34	Crab
33	Bananas	33	Sweet potatoes
30	Blackberries	25	Beets
25	Broccoli	24	Cauliflower
23	Carrots	22	Celery
21	Beef	20	Asparagus
19	Chicken	18	Pepper, green
17	Winter squash	16	Cantaloupe
16	Eggplant	14	Tomato
13	Cabbage	13	Grapes
13	Milk	13	Pineapple
13	Mushrooms	12	Onions
11	Oranges	11	Iceberg lettuce
9	Plums		

PHOSPHORUS

I.U. per
100-gram (3½ oz) portion

I.U. per
100-gram (3½ oz) portion

1753	Brewer's yeast	1276	Wheat bran
1144	Pumpkin and squash seeds	1118	Wheat germ
		837	Sunflower seeds
693	Brazil nuts	592	Sesame seeds, hulled
554	Soybeans, dried	504	Almonds
478	Cheddar cheese	457	Pinto beans, dried
409	Peanuts	400	Wheat
380	English walnuts	376	Rye Grain
373	Cashews	352	Beef liver
338	Scallops	311	Millet
290	Barley, pearled	289	Pecans
267	Dulse	240	Kelp
239	Chicken	221	Brown rice
202	Garlic	175	Crab
152	Cottage cheese	150	Beef or lamb
119	Lentils, cooked	116	Mushrooms
116	Fresh peas	111	Sweet corn
101	Raisins	93	Milk

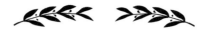

88	Globe artichoke	87	Yogurt
80	Brussels sprouts	79	Prunes, dried
78	Broccoli	77	Figs, dried
69	Yams	67	Soybean sprouts
64	Mung bean sprouts	63	Dates
63	Parsley	62	Asparagus
59	Bamboo shoots	56	Cauliflower
53	Potato, with skin	44	Green beans
44	Pumpkin	42	Avocado
40	Beet greens	39	Swiss chard
38	Winter squash	36	Carrots
36	Onions	35	Red cabbage
51	Spinach	33	Beets
31	Radishes	29	Summer squash
28	Celery	27	Cucumber
27	Tomatoes	26	Bananas
26	Persimmon	26	Eggplant
26	Lettuce	24	Nectarines
22	Raspberries	20	Grapes
20	Oranges	205	Eggs
17	Olives	16	Cantaloupe
10	Apples	8	Pineapple

SODIUM

I.U. per
100-gram (3½ oz) portion

I.U. per
100-gram (3½ oz) portion

3007	Kelp	2400	Green olives
2132	Salt (1 teaspoon)	1428	Dill pickles
1319	Soy sauce (1 tablespoon)	828	Ripe olives
747	Sauerkraut	700	Cheddar cheese
265	Scallops	229	Cottage cheese
210	Lobster	147	Swiss chard
130	Beet greens	130	Buttermilk
126	Celery	122	Eggs
110	Cod	71	Spinach
70	Lamb	65	Pork

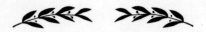

64	Chicken		60	Beef
60	Beets		60	Sesame seeds
52	Watercress		50	Whole milk
49	Turnips		47	Carrots
47	Yogurt		45	Parsley
43	Artichoke		34	Dried figs
30	Lentils, dried		30	Sunflower seeds
27	Raisins		26	Red cabbage
19	Garlic		19	White beans
15	Broccoli		15	Mushrooms
13	Cauliflower		10	Onions
10	Sweet Potatoes		9	Brown rice
9	Lettuce		6	Cucumber
5	Peanuts		4	Avocado
3	Tomatoes		2	Eggplant

POTASSIUM

I.U. per 100-gram ($3^1/_2$ oz) portion			I.U. per 100-gram ($3^1/_2$ oz) portion	
8060	Dulse		5273	Kelp
920	Sunflower seeds		827	Wheat germ
773	Almonds		763	Raisins
727	Parsley		715	Brazil nuts
674	Peanuts		648	Dates
640	Figs, dried		604	Avocado
603	Pecans		600	Yams
550	Swiss chard		540	Soybeans, cooked
529	Garlic		470	Spinach
450	English walnuts		430	Millet
416	Beans, cooked		414	Mushrooms
407	Potatoes, with skin		382	Broccoli
370	Bananas		370	Meats
369	Winter squash		366	Chicken
341	Carrots		341	Celery
322	Radishes		295	Cauliflower
282	Watercress		278	Asparagus

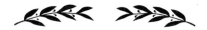

268	Red cabbage	264	Lettuce
251	Cantaloupe	249	Lentils, cooked
244	Tomatoes	243	Sweet potatoes
234	Papaya	214	Eggplant
213	Peppers, green	208	Beets
202	Peaches	202	Summer squash
200	Oranges	199	Raspberries
191	Cherries	164	Strawberries
162	Grapefruit juice	158	Grapes
157	Onions	146	Pineapple
144	Milk	141	Lemon juice
130	Pears	129	Eggs
110	Apples	100	Watermelon
70	Brown rice, cooked		

IRON

I.U. per 100-gram (3½ oz) portion		I.U. per 100-gram (3½ oz) portion	
100.3	Kelp	17.3	Brewer's yeast
16.1	Blackstrap molasses	14.9	Wheat bran
11.2	Pumpkin and squash seeds	9.4	Wheat germ
		8.8	Beef liver
7.1	Sunflower seeds	6.8	Millet
6.2	Parsley	6.1	Clam
4.7	Almond	3.9	Dried prunes
3.8	Cashews	3.7	Bccf, lean
3.5	Raisins	3.4	Jerusalem artichokes
3.4	Brazil nuts	3.3	Beet greens
3.2	Swiss chard	3.1	Dandelion greens
3.1	English walnuts	3.0	Dates
2.9	Pork	2.7	Cooked dry beans
2.4	Sesame seeds, hulled	2.4	Pecans
2.3	Eggs	2.1	Lentils
2.1	Peanuts	1.9	Lamb
1.9	Tofu	1.8	Green peas
1.6	Brown rice	1.6	Ripe olives

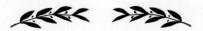

1.5	Chicken	1.3	Mung bean sprouts
1.2	Salmon	1.1	Broccoli
1.1	Currants	1.1	Whole wheat bread
1.1	Cauliflower	1.0	Cheddar cheese
1.0	Strawberries	1.0	Asparagus
0.9	Blackberries	0.8	Red cabbage
0.8	Pumpkin	0.8	Mushroom
0.7	Bananas	0.7	Beets
0.7	Carrots	0.7	Eggplant
0.7	Sweet potatoes	0.6	Avocado
0.6	Figs	0.6	Potatoes
0.6	Corn	0.5	Pineapple
0.5	Nectarines	0.5	Winter squash
0.5	Brown rice, cooked	0.5	Tomatoes
0.4	Oranges	0.4	Cherries
0.4	Summer squash	0.3	Papaya
0.3	Celery	0.3	Cottage Cheese
0.3	Apples		

COPPER

| I.U. per | | I.U. per | |
100-gram ($3^1/_2$ oz) portion		100-gram ($3^1/_2$ oz) portion	
13.7	Oysters	2.3	Brazil nuts
2.1	Soy lecithin	1.4	Almonds
1.3	Hazelnuts	1.3	Walnuts
1.3	Pecans	1.2	Split peas, dry
1.1	Beef liver	0.8	Buckwheat
0.8	Peanuts	0.7	Cod liver oil
0.7	Lamb chops	0.5	Sunflower oil
0.4	Butter	0.4	Rye grain
0.4	Pork loin	0.4	Barley
0.4	Gelatin	0.3	Shrimp
0.3	Olive oil	0.3	Clams
0.3	Carrots	0.3	Coconut
0.3	Garlic	0.2	Millet

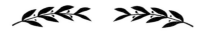

0.2	Whole wheat	0.2	Chicken
0.2	Eggs	0.2	Corn oil
0.2	Ginger root	0.2	Molasses
0.2	Turnips	0.1	Green peas
0.1	Papaya	0.1	Apples

Black pepper, thyme, paprika, bay leaves, and active dry yeast are also high in copper.

MANGANESE

I.U. per 100-gram (3½ oz) portion		I.U. per 100-gram (3½ oz) portion	
3.5	Pecans	2.8	Brazil nuts
2.5	Almonds	1.8	Barley
1.3	Rye	1.3	Buckwheat
1.3	Split peas, dry	1.1	Whole wheat
0.16	Carrots	0.15	Broccoli
0.14	Brown rice	0.14	Whole wheat bread
0.13	Swiss cheese	0.13	Corn
0.11	Cabbage	0.10	Peaches
0.8	Walnuts	0.8	Fresh spinach
0.7	Peanuts	0.6	Oats
0.5	Raisins	0.5	Turnip greens
0.5	Rhubarb	0.4	Beet greens
0.3	Brussels sprouts	0.3	Oatmeal
0.2	Cornmeal	0.2	Millet
0.19	Gorgonzola cheese	0.09	Butter
0.06	Tangerines	0.06	Peas
0.05	Eggs	0.04	Beets
0.04	Coconut	0.03	Apples
0.03	Oranges	0.03	Pears
0.03	Lamb chops	0.03	Pork chops
0.03	Cantaloupe	0.03	Tomatoes
0.02	Milk	0.02	Chicken breasts
0.02	Green beans	0.02	Apricots

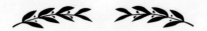

0.01	Beef liver	0.01	Scallops
0.01	Halibut	0.01	Cucumbers

Cloves, ginger, thyme, bay leaves, and tea are also high in manganese.

ZINC

I.U. per 100-gram (3½ oz) portion		I.U. per 100-gram (3½ oz) portion	
148.7	Fresh oysters	6.8	Ginger root
5.6	Ground round steak	5.3	Lamb chops
4.5	Pecans	4.2	Split peas, dry
4.2	Brazil nuts	3.9	Beef liver
3.5	Nonfat dry milk	3.5	Egg yolk
3.2	Whole wheat	3.2	Rye
3.2	Oats	3.2	Peanuts
3.1	Lima beans	3.1	Soy lecithin
3.1	Almonds	3.0	Walnuts
2.9	Sardines	2.6	Chicken
2.5	Buckwheat	2.4	Hazel nuts
1.9	Clams	1.7	Anchovies
1.7	Tuna	1.7	Haddock
1.6	Green peas	1.5	Shrimp
1.2	Turnips	0.9	Parsley
0.9	Potatoes	0.6	Garlic
0.5	Carrots	0.5	Whole wheat bread
0.4	Black beans	0.4	Raw milk
0.4	Pork chops	0.4	Corn
0.3	Grape juice	0.3	Olive oil
0.3	Cauliflower	0.2	Spinach
0.2	Cabbage	0.2	Lentils
0.2	Butter	0.2	Lettuce
0.1	Cucumber	0.1	Yams
0.1	Tangerines	0.1	String beans

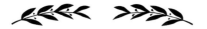

CHROMIUM

The values listed below show the total chromium content of these foods, and do not indicate the amount that may be biologically active as the Glucose Tolerance Factor (GTF). Those foods marked with an * are high in GTF.

I.U. per 100-gram (3½ oz) portion		I.U. per 100-gram (3½ oz) portion	
112	Brewer's yeast*	57	Beef round
55	Calf liver*	42	Whole wheat bread*
38	Wheat bran	30	Rye bread
30	Fresh chili	26	Oysters
24	Potatoes	23	Wheat germ
19	Peppers, green	16	Hen's eggs
15	Chicken	14	Apples
13	Butter	13	Parsnips
12	Cornmeal	12	Lamb chop
11	Scallops	11	Swiss cheese
10	Bananas	10	Spinach
10	Pork chop	9	Carrots
8	Navy beans, dry	7	Shrimp
7	Lettuce	5	Oranges
5	Lobster tails	5	Blueberries
4	Green beans	4	Cabbage
4	Mushrooms	3	Beer
3	Strawberries	1	Milk

SELENIUM

I.U. per 100-gram (3½ oz) portion		I.U. per 100-gram (3½ oz) portion	
144	Butter	141	Smoked herring
123	Smelts	111	Wheat germ
103	Brazil nuts	89	Apple cider vinegar

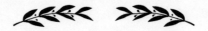

77	Scallops		66	Barley
66	Whole wheat bread		65	Lobster
63	Bran		59	Shrimps
57	Red swiss chard		56	Oats
55	Clams		51	King crab
49	Oysters		48	Milk
43	Cod		39	Brown rice
34	Top round steak		30	Lamb
27	Turnips		26	Molasses
25	Garlic		24	Barley
19	Orange juice		19	Gelatin
19	Beer		18	Beef liver
18	Lamb chop		18	Egg yolk
12	Mushrooms		12	Chicken
10	Swiss cheese		5	Cottage cheese
5	Wine		4	Radishes
4	Grape juice		3	Pecans
2	Hazelnuts		2	Almonds
2	Green beans		2	Kidney beans
2	Onions		2	Carrots
2	Cabbage		1	Oranges

IODINE

I.U. per 100-gram (3½ oz) portion			I.U. per 100-gram (3½ oz) portion	
90	Clams		65	Shrimp
62	Haddock		56	Halibut
50	Oysters		50	Salmon
37	Sardines, canned		19	Beef liver
16	Pineapple		16	Tuna, canned
14	Eggs		11	Peanuts
11	Whole wheat bread		11	Cheddar Cheese
10	Pork		10	Lettuce
9	Spinach		9	Green peppers
9	Butter		7	Milk

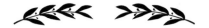

6	Cream	6	Cottage cheese
6	Beef	3	Lamb
3	Raisins		

NICKEL

I.U. per 100-gram (3½ oz) portion		I.U. per 100-gram (3½ oz) portion	
700	Soybeans, dry	500	Beans, dry
410	Soy flour	310	Lentils
250	Split peas	175	Green peas
153	Green beans	150	Oats
132	Walnuts	122	Hazelnuts
100	Buckwheat	90	Barley
90	Corn	90	Parsley
38	Whole wheat	35	Spinach
30	Fish	27	Cucumbers
26	Liver	25	Rye bread
25	Pork	25	Carrots
24	Eggs	22	Cabbage
20	Tomatoes	20	Onions
16	Potatoes	16	Beef
16	Apricots	16	Oranges
15	Cheese	15	Watermelon
14	Lettuce	13	Apples
12	Whole wheat bread	12	Beets
12	Pears	8	Grapes
8	Radishes	6	Pine nuts
6	Lamb	3	Milk

MOLYBDENUM

I.U. per 100-gram (3½ oz) portion		I.U. per 100-gram (3½ oz) portion	
155	Lentils	135	Beef liver
130	Split peas	120	Cauliflower
110	Green peas	109	Brewer's yeast

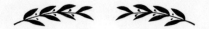

100	Spinach	100	Wheat germ
77	Beef kidney	75	Brown rice
70	Garlic	60	Oats
53	Eggs	50	Rye bread
45	Corn	42	Barley
40	Fish	36	Whole wheat
32	Whole wheat bread	32	Chicken
31	Cottage cheese	30	Beef
30	Potatoes	25	Onions
25	Peanuts	25	Coconut
25	Pork	24	Lamb
21	Green beans	19	Crab
19	Molasses	16	Cantaloupe
14	Apricots	10	Raisins
10	Butter	7	Strawberries
5	Carrots	5	Cabbage
3	Whole milk	1	Goat's milk

VANADIUM

I.U. per 100-gram (3½ oz) portion		I.U. per 100-gram (3½ oz) portion	
100	Buckwheat	80	Parsley
70	Soybeans	64	Safflower oil
42	Eggs	41	Sunflower seed oil
35	Oats	30	Olive oil
15	Sunflower seeds	15	Corn
14	Green beans	11	Peanut oil
10	Carrots	10	Cabbage
10	Garlic	6	Tomatoes
5	Radishes	5	Onions
5	Whole wheat	4	Lobster
4	Beets	3	Apples
2	Plums	2	Lettuce
2	Millet		

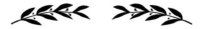

BAD FOOD

The following foods contain large amounts of sodium chloride, added during processing, and should generally be avoided.

Canned or frozen vegetables
Cured, smoked,
or canned meats
Commercial peanut butter
Potato chips, corn chips, etc.
Processed cheeses
Luncheon meats
Salted nuts

Packaged spice mixes
Bouillon cubes
Canned fish
Salted crackers
Canned or packaged soups
Commercial salad dressings
Meat tenderizers

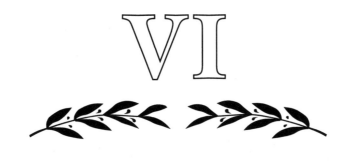

VI

SOURCES OF INFORMATION
ON GOOD NUTRITION

SOURCES OF INFORMATION ON GOOD NUTRITION

❦

While writing this book, I have consulted the following list of publications. Some of the authors are named in the book as the sources of my information. Readers may find this bibliography useful for learning more about good nutrition.

Abou-Saleh, M.T., and A. Coppen. "The Biology of Folate in Depression: Implications for Nutritional Hypotheses of the Psychoses." *Journal of Psychiatric Research,* 20: 91-101, 1986.

Agnew N., and A. Hoffer. "Nicotinic Acid Modified Lysergic Acid Diethylamide Psychosis." *Journal of Mental Science,* 101: 12-27, 1955.

Altschul R., A. Hoffer, and J.D. Stephen. "Influence of Nicotinic Acid on Serum Cholesterol in Man." *Archives of Biochemistry and Biophysics,* 54: 558-559, 1955.

Anderson, J., J. Brosnan, J. Hoffer, J. Johnston, L. Leiter, G.S. Pandey, and N. Sayem. *Report of the Expert Advisory Committee on Amino Acids.* Ottawa, ON: Health and Welfare, Canada, 1990.

Beasley, J.D., and J.J. Swift. *The Kellogg Report. The Impact of Nutrition, Environment & Lifestyle on the Health of Americans.* Annandale-on-Hudson, NY: The Institute of Health Policy and Practice, The Bard College Center, 1989.

Benjamin, H. *et al.* "Inhibition of Benzo[a]pyrene-induced Mouse Forestomach Neoplasia by Dietary Soy Sauce."

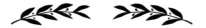

Cancer Research, 51: 2940-2943, 1991.

Benjamin, H. *et al.* "Reduction of Benzo[a]pyrene induced Forestomach Neoplasms in Mice Given Nitrite and Dietary Soy Sauce." *Food Chemical Toxicology,* 26: 671-678, 1988.

Benton, D., and R. Cook. "The Impact of Selenium Supplementation on Mood." *Biological Psychiatry,* 29: 1092-1098, 1991.

Benton, D. "Dietary Sugar, Hyperactivity and Cognitive Functioning: A Methodological Review." *Journal of Applied Nutrition,* 41: 13-22, 1989.

Benton, D., and R. Cook. "Vitamin and Mineral Supplements Improve the Intelligence Scores and Concentration of Six-Year-Old Children." *Personality and Individual Differences,* 12: 1151-1158, 1991.

Boman, B. "L-tryptophan: A Rational Anti-Depressant and a Natural Hypnotic ?" *Australian and New Zealand Journal of Psychiatry,* 22: 83-97, 1988.

Braverman, E.R., and C.C. Pfeiffer. *The Healing Nutrients Within.* New Canaan, CT: Keats Publishing, 1987.

Burke, K.E., G.F. Combs, Jr., E.G. Gross, K.C. Bhuyan, and H. Abu-Libdeh. "The Effects of Topical and Oral L-selenomethionine on Pigmentation and Skin Cancer Induced by Ultraviolet Irradiation." *Nutrition and Cancer,* 17: 123-137, 1992.

Butterworth, C.E., K.D. Hatch, M. Macaluso, P. Cole, H.E. Sauberlich, Soong Seng-Jaw, M. Borst, and V.V. Baker. "Folate Deficiency and Cervical Dysplasia." *Journal of the American Medical Association,* 267: 528-533, 1992.

Caldwell, A.E. *Origins of Psychopharmacology from CPZ to LSD.* Springfield, IL: C.C. Thomas, 1970.

Campbell, J.D. "Hair Analysis: A Diagnostic Tool for Measuring Mineral Status in Humans." *Journal of Orthomolecular Psychiatry,* 14: 276-280, 1985.

Campbell, J.D. "Hair Tissue Mineral Analysis: A Review." *Townsend Letter for Doctors,* 118: 436-444, May, 1993.

Canner, P.L., K.G. Berge, N.K. Wenger, J. Stamler, L. Friedman, R.J. Prineas, and W. Friedewald. "Fifteen Year Mortality in Coronary Drug Project Patients: Long Term Benefit With Niacin." *Journal of the American College of Cardiology,* 8: 1245-1255, 1986.

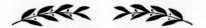

Challem, J. "Too Much Iron . . . or Too Little Vitamin E." *The Nutrition Reporter,* 4: 1 & 4, 1993.

Cheraskin, E., W.M. Ringsdorf, and E.L. Sisley. *The Vitamin C Connection.* New York: Harper and Row, 1983.

Cheraskin, E., W.M. Ringsdorf, and E.L. Sisley. *The Vitamin C Controversy: Questions and Answers.* Wichita, KS: Bio-Communications Press, 1988.

Cleave, T.L. *The Saccharine Disease.* New Canaan, CT: Keats Publishing, 1975.

Cleave, T.L., G.D. Campbell, and N.S. Painter. *Diabetes, Coronary Thrombosis and the Saccharine Disease.* Bristol, England: Wright & Sons Ltd, 1960.

Colborn, T. and C. Clement. *Chemically-induced Alterations in Sexual and Functional Development: The Wildlife/Human Connection.* Advances in Modern Environmental Toxicology, Vol. 21. Princeton, NJ: Princeton Scientific Publishing, 1992.

Commentary. "Oral Cobalamin for Pernicious Anemia: Medicine's Best Kept Secret?" *Journal of the American Medical Association,* 265: 94-95, 1991.

Cott, A. "Orthomolecular Approach to the Treatment of Learning Disabilities. *Journal of Orthomolecular Psychiatry,* 3: 95-105, 1971.

Cott, A. *Dr. Cotts Help for Your Learning Disabled Child.* New York, NY: Times Books, 1985.

Cott, A. "Orthomolecular Approach to the Treatment of Children with Behavioral Disorders and Learning Disabilities." *Journal of Applied Nutrition,* 25: 15-24, 1973.

Cromwell, P.E., B.R. Abadie, J.D. Stephens, and M. Kyler. "Hair Mineral Analysis: Biochemical Imbalances and Violent Criminal Behavior." *Psychological Reports,* 64: 259-266, 1989.

Crook. W.G. *Can Your Child Read? Is He Hyperactive?* Jackson, TN: Professional Books, 1977.

Crook. W.G. *Detecting Your Hidden Allergies.* Jackson, TN: Professional Books, 1988.

Crook. W.G. *Solving the Puzzle of Your Hard-to-Raise Child.* New York, NY: Random House, 1987.

Cutler, P. "Iron Overload in Psychiatric Illness." *American*

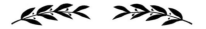

Journal of Psychiatry, 148: 1, 1991.

Davis, D.R. "The Harrell Study and Seven Follow-Up Studies: A Brief Review." *Journal of Orthomolecular Medicine,* 2: 111-115, 1987.

Di Cyan, E. *Vitamin E and Aging.* New York, NY: Pyramid Books, 1972.

Egger, J., J. Wilson, C. M. Carter, M.W. Turner, and J.F. Soothill. "Is Migraine Food Allergy? A Double Blind Controlled Trial of Oligoantigenic Diet Treatments." *Lancet,* 2: 865-868, 1983.

Eisenberg, D.M., R.C. Kessler, C. Foster, F.E. Norlock, D.R. Calkins, and T.L. Delbanco. "Unconventional Medicine in The United States." *New England Journal of Medicine,* 328: 246-252, 1993.

Erasmus, Udo. *Fats and Oils,* Vancouver, BC: Alive, 1986.

Finn, R. "Food Allergy — Fact or Fiction: A Review." *Journal of the Royal Society of Medicine,* 85: 560-563, 1992.

Finnegan, J. *The Facts about Fats.* Malibu, CA: Elysian Arts, 1992.

Foster, H.D. "Fluoride and Its Antagonists: Implications for Human Health." *Journal of Orthomolecular Medicine,* 8: 149-53, 1993.

Foster, H.D. *Health, Disease and the Environment.* Boca Raton, FL: CRC Press, 1992.

Freeland-Graves, J.H. "Manganese: An Essential Nutrient for Humans." *Nutrition Today,* 13 -19, Nov/Dec, 1988.

Gaby, A.R. & J.V. Wright. *Nutrients and Bone Health.* xxxxx Wright/Gaby Nutrition Institute, August 1988.

Galler, J.R. *Human Nutrition.* New York, NY: Plenum Press, 1984.

Gerrard, J.W. *Understanding Allergies.* Springfield, IL: C. C. Thomas, 1973.

Gray, A.S. "Fluoridation: Time for a New Base Line?" *Journal of the Canadian Dental Association,* 10: 763-765, 1987.

Gray, C. "British MD's Face Growing Pressure from Alternative Medicine, Government." *Canadian Medical Association Journal,* 143: 132-143, 1990.

Goodhart, R.S. and M.E. Shils. *Modern Nutrition in Health and Disease.* Philadelphia, PA: Lea & Febiger, 1974.

Hackman, R.M. "Chromium and Cholesterol." *Townsend Letter for Doctors,* 744 -748, October, 1991.

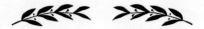

Hahn, L.J., R Kloiber, M.J. Vimy, Y. Takahashi, and F.L. Lorscheider. "Dental Silver Tooth Fillings: A Source of Mercury Exposure Revealed by Whole-Body Image Scan and Tissue Analysis." *Journal of the Federation of American Societies for Experimental Biology,* 3: 2641-2646, 1989.

Hall, Rose Hume. *Food for Naught: The Decline in Nutrition.* New York, NY: Harper and Row, 1974.

Hanson, M. "Amalgam — Hazards in Your Teeth." *Journal of Orthomolecular Psychiatry,* 12: 194-201, 1983.

Hattersley, J.G. "The Answer to Crib Death." *Journal of Orthomolecular Medicine,* 8: 229-45, 1993.

Heaney, R. "Editorial." *New England Journal Medicine,* 328: 503-505, 1993.

Hemingway, D.C. "Good Nutrition Lowers Health Care Costs." *Journal of Orthomolecular Medicine,* 7: 67-71, 1992.

Henkin, Y., K.C. Johnson, and J.P. Segrest. "Rechallenge with Crystalline Niacin after Drug-Induced Hepatitis from Sustained-Release Niacin." *Journal of American Medical Association,* 264: 241-243, 1990.

Herbert, V. and E. Jacobs. "Destruction of Vitamin B-12 by Ascorbic Acid." *Journal of the American Medical Association,* 230: 241-242, 1974.

Hileman, B. "Fluoridation of Water." *Chemical & Engineering News,* 26-42, August 1, 1988.

Hippchen, L.J. "An Exploratory Study of the Use of Nutritional Approaches in the Treatment of Suicide Prone Persons." *Journal of Orthomolecular Psychiatry,* 10: 147, 1981.

Hippchen, L.J. *Ecologic, Biochemical Approach to Treatment of Delinquents and Criminals.* New York, NY: Van Nostrand Reinhold Co., 1978.

Hoffer, A. "A Vitamin B-3 Dependent Family." *Schizophrenia,* 3: 41-46, 1971.

Hoffer, A. "Ascorbic Acid and Kidney Stones." *Canadian Medical Association Journal,* 132: 320, 1985.

Hoffer, A. "Children With Learning and Behavioral Disorders." *Journal of Orthomolecular Psychiatry,* 5: 228-230, 1976.

Hoffer, A. "Chronic Schizophrenic Patients Treated Ten Years

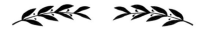

or More." *Journal of Orthomolecular Medicine*, 8: 7-37, 1994.

Hoffer, A. *Common Questions on Schizophrenia and Their Answers.* New Canaan, CT: Keats Publishing, 1988.

Hoffer, A. "Five California Schizophrenics." *Journal of Schizophrenia*, 1: 209-220, 1967.

Hoffer, A. "Hong Kong Veterans Study." *Journal of Orthomolecular Psychiatry*, 3: 34-36, 1974.

Hoffer, A. "Hyperactivity, Allergy and Megavitamins." *Canadian Medical Association Journal*, 111: 905-907, 1974.

Hoffer, A. *Niacin Therapy in Psychiatry.* Springfield, IL: C. C. Thomas, 1962.

Hoffer, A. *Orthomolecular Medicine for Physicians.* New Canaan, CT: Keats Publishing, 1989.

Hoffer A. "Orthomolecular Nutrition at the Zoo." *Journal of Orthomolecular Psychiatry*, 12: 116-128, 1983.

Hoffer, A. "Safety, Side Effects and Relative Lack of Toxicity of Nicotinic Acid and Nicotinamide." *Schizophrenia*, 1: 78-87, 1969.

Hoffer, A. *Vitamin B-3 (Niacin) Update. New Roles For a Key Nutrient in Diabetes, Cancer, Heart Disease and Other Major Health Problems.* New Canaan, CT: Keats Publishing, 1990.

Hoffer, A. "Vitamin and Mineral Supplements Increase Intelligence." *Nutrition Health Review*, Fall, 1989.

Hoffer, A. "Vitamin B-3 Dependent Child." *Schizophrenia*, 3: 107-113, 1971.

Hoffer, A., and H. Osmond. *The Hallucinogens.* New York, NY: Academic Press, 1967.

Hoffer, A. and L. Pauling. "Hardin Jones Biostatistical Analysis of Mortality Data for Cohorts of Cancer Patients with a Large Fraction Surviving at the Termination of the Study and a Comparison of Survival Times of Cancer Patients Receiving Large Regular Oral Doses of Vitamin C and Other Nutrients with Similar Patients not Receiving those Doses." *Journal of Orthomolecular Medicine*, 5: 143-154, 1990.

Hoffer, A. and M. Walker. *Smart Nutrients.* Garden City Park, NY: Avery Publishing Group, 1994.

Hoffer, A. and M. Walker. *Orthomolecular Nutrition.* New

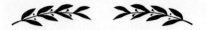

Canaan, CT: Keats Publishing, 1978.

Hoffer A., H.Osmond, M.J. Callbeck, and I. Kahan. "Treatment of Schizophrenia with Nicotinic Acid and Nicotinamide." *Journal of Clinical and Experimental Psychopathology*, 18: 131-158, 1957.

Hoffer, A., H. Osmond, and J. Smythies, "Schizophrenia: A New Approach. II. Results of a Year's Research." *Journal of Mental Science*, 100: 29-45, 1954.

Horrobin, D.F. "Schizophrenia as a Prostaglandin Deficiency Disease." *Lancet*, 1: 936-937, 1977.

Horrobin, D.F. *Clinical Uses for Essential Fatty Acids*. St. Albans: Eden Press, 1983.

Horrobin, D.F. "Gamma Linolenic Acid: An Intermediate in Essential Fatty Acid Metabolism with Potential as an Ethical Pharmaceutical and as a Food." *Review of Contemporary Pharmacotherapy*, 1: 1-45, 1990.

Horrobin, D.F., M. Oka, and M.S. Manku. "The Regulation of Prostaglandin E 1 Formation: A Candidate for One of the Fundamental Mechanisms Involved in the Actions of Vitamin C." *Medical Hypothesis*, 5: 849-858, 1979.

Hughes, J. and R.W. Norman. "Diet and Calcium Stones." *Canadian Medical Association Journal*, 146: 137-142, 1992.

Huggins, H.A. "Mercury: A Factor in Mental Disease."*Journal of Orthomolecular Psychiatry*, 11: 3-16, 1982.

Johnstone, E.C. *et al.* "Disabilities and Circumstances of Schizophrenic Patients — A Follow-Up Study." *The British Journal of Psychiatry*, 159, Supplement 13, 1991.

Kaplan, B.J., N. McNicol, R.A. Conte, and H.K. Moghadam. "Dietary Replacement in Preschool-Aged Hyperactive Boys."*Pediatrics* 83: 7-17, 1989.

Kaufman, W. *Common Form of Niacinamide Deficiency Disease: Aniacinamidosis*. New Haven, CT: Yale University Press, 1943.

Kotkas,L. "B$_{12}$ and Folic Acid in Treatment of Some Psychiatric Illnesses." Annual Meeting of the Canadian Schizophrenia Foundation, June 4th, 1978.

Krilanovic, N. *No Sugar Added*. Santa Barbara: November Books, 1982.

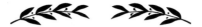

Kunin, R.A. "Manganese and Niacin in the Treatment of Drug-Induced Dyskinesias." *Journal of Orthomolecular Psychiatry,* 5: 4-27, 1976.

Lowry, F. "Prescription of Health." Report to the Pharmaceutical Inquiry of Ontario, July 1990.

Machlin, L.J. "Introduction." *Annals of the New York Academy of Sciences,* 669: 1-6, 1992

Mandell, M. and L.W. Scanlon. *Dr. Mandell's 5 Day Allergy Relief System.* New York, NY: Thomas Y. Crowell, 1979.

Marlowe, M., D. Medeiros, C. Moon, J. Errera, and L. Medeiros. "Hair Minerals, Diet and Behavior of Prader-Willi Syndrome Youth." *Journal of Orthomolecular Medicine,* 2: 146-153, 1987.

Marlowe, M., J. Errera, J. Stellern, and D. Beck. "Lead and Mercury Levels in Emotionally Disturbed Children." *Journal of Orthomolecular Science,* 12: 260-267, 1983.

Martin, W. "Soy and Breast Cancer." *Townsend Letter for Doctors,* April 328-329, 1993.

McLachlan, D.R.C., T.P Kruck, W.J. Lukiw, and S.S. Krishnan. "Would Decreased Aluminum Ingestion Reduce the Incidence of Alzheimers Disease?" *Canadian Medical Association Journal,* 145: 793-804, 1991.

McCarron, D.A., C.D.Morris, H.J. Henry, and J.L. Stanton. "Blood Pressure and Nutrient Intake in the United States." *Science,* 224: 1392-1398, 1984.

Mitchell, J. "Dairy Tales. There's More Myth than Truth to the Fears Fueling the Growing Dairy Phobia." *Globe and Mail,* 1993.

Moore, R.D. and G. D. Webb, *The K Factor.* New York, NY: Macmillan Publishing, 1986.

Moss, W.W. *Cancer Therapy. The Independent Consumers Guide to Non-Toxic Treatment & Prevention.* New York, NY: Equinox Press, 1992.

Mullin, G.E., J.K.Greenson, and M.C. Mitchell. "Fulminant Hepatic Failure after Ingestion of Sustained-Release Nicotinic Acid." *Annals of Internal Medicine,* 111: 253-255, 1989.

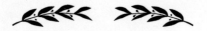

Newbold, H. L. *Mega Nutrients for Your Nerves*. New York, NY: Peter Wyden Publishing, 1975.

Nolan, K.R. "Copper Toxicity Syndrome." *Journal of Orthomolecular Psychiatry*, 12: 270-282, 1983.

Oski, Frank A. *Don't Drink Your Milk: The Frightening New Medical Facts about the Worlds Most Overrated Nutrient*. Syracuse, NY: Mollica Press Ltd. 1977.

Pauling, L. "Are Recommended Daily Allowances for Vitamin C Adequate?" *Proceedings of the National Academy of Sciences USA*, 71: 4442-4446, 1974.

Pauling, L. *How to Live Longer and Feel Better.* N Y: W. H. Freeman, 1986.

Pauling, L. "Orthomolecular Psychiatry." *Science,* 160: 265-271, 1968.

Pauling, L. *Vitamin C and the Common Cold*. San Francisco: W.H. Freeman, 1970.

Pfeiffer, C.C. *Mental and Elemental Nutrients*. New Canaan, CT: Keats Publishing, 1975.

Pfeiffer, C.C. *Zinc and Other Micro-Nutrients*. New Canaan, CT: Keats Publishing, 1978.

Pfeiffer, C.C. and S. LaMola. "Zinc and Manganese in the Schizophrenias." *Journal of Orthomolecular Psychiatry*, 12: 215-234, 1983.

Passwater, R.A. "L-glutamine: The Surprising Brain Fuel." *Health Express*, 2: 8 -11, 1981.

Petersdorf, R.G. *et al. Harrisons Principles of Internal Medicine*. 10th edition. New York, NY: McGraw Hill, 1983.

Phillpott, W.H. "Ecologic, Orthomolecular and Behavioral Contributors to Psychiatry. " *Orthomolecular Psychiatry*, 3: 356-370, 1968.

Phillpott, W.H. "Maladaptive Reactions to Frequently Used Foods and Commonly Met Chemicals and Chronic Factors in Many Chronic Physical and Chronic Emotional Illnesses." *A Physicians Handbook on Orthomolecular Medicine*. Ed. R. J.Williams and D. K. Kalita. New Canaan, CT: Keats Publishing, 1979.

Philpott, W.H. and D.K. Kalita. *Brain Allergies: The Psychonutrient Connection*. New Canaan, CT: Keats Publishing, 1980.

Philpott, W.H. and D.K. Kalita. *Brain Allergies: The Psychonutrient Connection*. New Canaan, CT: Keats Publishing, 1980.

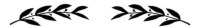

Pleva, J. "Mercury Poisoning from Dental Amalgam." *Journal of Orthomolecular Psychiatry,* 12: 184-193, 1983.

Prasad, A.S. *Trace Elements in Human Health and Disease; Vol 1: Zinc and Copper.* New York, NY: Academic Press, 1976.

Randolph, T.G. and R.W. Moss. *An Alternative Approach to Allergies.* New York, NY: Harper and Row, 1980.

Rapp, D. *Allergies and the Hyperactive Child.* New York, NY: Cornerstone Library, 1979.

Rath, M. and L. Pauling. "Solution to the Puzzle of Human Cardiovascular Disease: Its Primary Cause Is Ascorbate Deficiency Leading to the Deposition of Lipoprotein(a) and Fibrinogen/Fibrin in the Vascular Wall. *Journal of Orthomolecular Medicine,* 6: 125-134, 1991.

Reed, B. *Food, Teens and Behavior.* Manitowoc, WI: Natural Press, 1983.

Reuler, J.B., V.C. Broudy, and T.G. Cooney. "Adult Scurvy." *Journal of American Medical Association,* 253: 805-807, 1985.

Richards, E. *Vitamin C and Cancer: Medicine or Politics?* London: Macmillan, 1991.

Riggs, L. *The Medical Post,* April 10, 1990.

Rimland, B. "Recent Research in Infantile Autism." *Journal of Operational Psychiatry,* 3: 35, 1972; *Autism Research Review International,* 7: No 2, 1993.

Rimland. B. "The Feingold Diet: An Assessment of the Reviews by Mattes, Kavale and Forness and Others." *Journal of Learning Disabilities,* 16: 331-333, 1983.

Rimland, B., E. Callaway, and P. Dreyfus. "The Effect of High Doses of Vitamin B-6 on Autistic Children: A Double Blind Crossover Study." *American Journal of Psychiatry,* 135: 472-475, 1978.

Rimm, E.B., M.J. Stampfer, A. Ascherio, E. Giovannucci, G.A. Colditz, and W.C. Willett. "Vitamin E Consumption and the Risk of Coronary Heart Disease in Men." *New England Journal Medicine,* 328: 1450-1456, 1993.

Rogers, L.L. and R.B. Pelton. "Effect of Glutamine on IQ Scores of Mentally Deficient Children." *Texas Reports on Biology and Medicine,* 15: 84-90, 1957.

Ross, H. *Fighting Depression.* New York, NY: Larchmont Books, 1975.

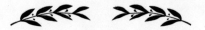

Rowen R. "Alaska Governor Appoints Alternative Doctor." *Health Action*, Winter 1992/1993.

Rudin, D.O. and C. Felix, *The Omega-3 Phenomenon*. New York, NY: Rawson Associates, 1987.

Sakimoto, K. "The Cause of the Eosinophilia-Myalgia Syndrome Associated with Tryptophan Use." *New England Journal of Medicine*, 323: 992-993, 1990.

Schauss, A.G. "Chromium Picolinate and Bariatric Medicine." *International Journal of Biosocial Medical Research*, 13: 152-1563, 1991.

Schauss, A.G. *Diet, Crime and Delinquency*. Berkeley, CA: Parker House, 1980.

Schauss, A.G. "Zinc Status and Eating Disorders." *International Journal of Biosocial Medical Research*, 13: 153-156, 1991.

Schoenthaler, S.J., W.E. Doraz, and J.A. Wakefield. "The Impact of a Low Food Additive and Sucrose Diet on Academic Performance in 803 New York City Public Schools." *International Journal of Biosocial Research*, 8: 185-195, 1986.

Shine, I. *Serendipity and St. Helena*. New York, NY: Pergamon Press, 1970.

Shriqui, C. "Issues Related to the Long-Term Treatment of Schizophrenia. *Schizophrenia Management*, 1: February, 1993.

Siblerund, R.L. "The Relationship between Mercury from Dental Amalgam and Mental Health." *American Journal of Psychotherapy*, 43: 575-587, 1989.

Simons, F.E.R., Z.H. Chad, H.A. Sampson, S.M. Tarlo, and R.K. Chandra. "Food Allergy and Intolerance: New Directions." *Annals of The Royal College of Physicians and Surgeons of Canada*, 26: 29-32, 1993.

Slagle, P. *The Way Up from Down*. New York, NY: Random House, 1987.

Smith, L. *Foods for Healthy Kids*. New York, NY: McGraw Hill, 1981.

Smith, M. "Canadian Tests Link Anorexia to Deficiency of Zinc in Diet." *Vancouver Sun*, February 27, 1993.

Soothill, J. "Food Intolerance." *The Practitioner*, 233: 596-602, 1989.

Stampfer, M.J., C.H. Hennekens, J. Manson, G.A. Colditz, B.

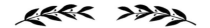

Rosner, and W.C. Willett. "Vitamin E Consumption and the Risk of Coronary Disease in Women." *New England Journal Medicine*, 328: 1444-1449, 1993.

Stone, I. "The Healing Factor: Vitamin C Against Disease." New York: Grosset and Dunlap, 1972.

Swank, R.L., and M.H. Pullen. *The Multiple Sclerosis Diet Book.* New York: Doubleday, 1977.

Truss, C.O. *The Missing Diagnosis.* Birmingham, AL: Self-Published, 1983.

Truss, C.O. "The Role of Candida Albicans in Human Illness." *Journal of Orthomolecular Psychiatry,* 10: 228-238, 1981.

Turkel, N, and I. Nusbaum. *Medical Treatment of Down's Syndrome and Genetic Diseases.* Southfield, MI: Ubiotica, 1985.

Turkel, H. "Medical Amelioration of Down's Syndrome Incorporating the Orthomolecular Approach. *Journal of Orthomolecular Psychiatry* , 4: 102-115, 1975.

Turkel, H., "Treatment of a Mucopolusaccharide Type of Storage Disease with the 'U' Series." *Journal of Orthomolecular Psychiatry,* 10: 239-248, 1981.

Urberg, M. and M.G. Zemel. "Evidence for Synergism between Chromium and Nicotinic Acid in the Control of Glucose Tolerance in Elderly Humans." *Metabolism,* 36: 896-899, 1987.

Vance, D.E., W.D. Ehmann, and W.R. Markesbery. "Trace Element Imbalances in Hair and Nails of Alzheimers Disease Patients." *Neurotoxicology,* 9: 197-208, 1988.

Waler, M.M. "Phosphates as a Cause of Hyperactivity. *" Health Express,* 2: 15 -17, 61, 1981.

Weber, C.W., G.W. Nelson, M. V. de Vaquera, and P.B. Pearson. "Trace Elements in Hair of Healthy and Malnourished Children. *Journal of Topical Pediatrics,* 36: 230-234, 1990.

Williams, R.J. *Alcoholism: The Nutritional Approach.* Austin, TX: University of Texas Press, 1958.

Young. S.N. "Tryptophan Availability in Humans: Effects on Mood and Behavior." *Nato ASI:* Series H20, 267-274, 1988.

Young. S.N. "Use of Tryptophan in Combination with Other Antidepressant Treatments: A Review. *Journal of Psychiatry and Neuroscience,* 16: 241-246, 1991.

Young, S.N. and A.M. Ghadirian. "Folic Acid and Psychopathology." *Progressive Neuro-Pyschopharmacology and*

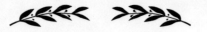

Biological Psychiatry, 13: 841-863, 1989.

Young, S.N., and K.L. Teff. "Tryptophan Availability: 5HT Synthesis and 5HT Function." *Progressive Neuro-Pyschopharm ocology & Biological Psychiatry,* 13: 373-379, 1989.

Zamm, A.V. "Candida Albicans Therapy: Is There Ever an End to It? Dental Mercury Removal: An Effective Adjunct." *Journal of Orthomolecular Medicine,* 1: 261-266, 1986.

Zamm, A.V. "Dental Mercury: A Factor that Aggravates and Induces Xenobiotic Intolerance." *Journal of Orthomolecular Medicine ,* 6: 67-78, 1991.

Zamm, A.V. "Removal of Dental Mercury: Often an Effective Treatment for the Very Sensitive Patient. *Journal of Orthomolecular Medicine,* 5: 138-42,1990.